D0867648

$19.95

Meeting the Challenge
of
Progressive Multiple Sclerosis

CLAYTON-LIBERTY TWP LIBRARY
Clayton, IN 46118

616.8
COYLE

S 020825

Meeting the Challenge

of

Pr~~~~~~~~~~~~~~~sis

616.8   S 020825
COYLE
          Coyle, Patricia

Meeting the challenge of
progressive multiple sclerosis

DATE DUE			
APR 29 2003			

The Stony ~~~~~~~~~~~~~~~~~~~~~~~~~~~~~~~~ Center

CLAYTON-LIBERTY TWP LIBRARY
Clayton, IN 46118

New York

Demos Medical Publishing, Inc., 386 Park Avenue South, New York, New York 10016

© 2001 by Demos Medical Publishing, Inc. All rights reserved. This book is protected by copyright. No part of it may be reproduced, stored in a retrieval system, or transmitted in any form or by any means, electronic, mechanical, photocopying, recording, or otherwise, without the prior written permission of the publisher.

Library of Congress Cataloging-in-Publication Data

Coyle, Patricia K.
   Meeting the challenge of progressive multiple sclerosis / Patricia Coyle, June Halper.
      p. cm.
   Includes bibliographical references and index.
   ISBN 1-88799-46-3 (alk. paper)
      1. Multiple sclerosis—Popular works.   I. Halper, June.   II. Title.

   RC377.C69 2001
   616.8'34—dc21

                                                                00-069370

Printed in Canada

Dedication

To my beloved parents—Eileen Jane and Daniel Edward Coyle
P.K.C.

To the memory of Edward I. Zurndorfer,
who met the challenges of progressive
MS with great courage and dignity
J.H.

Contents

Preface

With its variable disease course and wide array of symptoms, multiple sclerosis (MS) presents each individual with ongoing challenges. When confronted with signs of disease progression, these challenges are increased and intensified. It is important to acknowledge these problems both to yourself, to your family and loved ones, and to your health care providers. Once acknowledged, many of these problems can be resolved or at least managed with appropriate pharmacologic and nonpharmacologic interventions.

People with MS now have choices that can evolve into hope: hope for disease modification and symptom reduction, hope for a full and desired quality of life, and hope for future breakthroughs in research.

The important take-away message is that MS is no longer (as Dr. Labe Scheinberg used to say) "diagnose and adios." It is a complex disease that requires skilled and ongoing assessment, reassessment, and care. It is also a condition that one can live with and cope with successfully, given appropriate supports.

The new millennium brings with it the promise of new research advances and a greater understanding of neurologic diseases such as MS. The authors of this book hope that our readers will continue to seek appropriate health care for their condition, as well as identify and utilize services and programs available to those with chronic illness and disability. The wellness approach to progressive MS consists of weighing options and exploring possibilities, hoping and planning, and maintaining a sense of humor and a sense of wonder for possibilities and promise in life.

Acknowledgments

P.K.C. acknowledges the expert assistance of Isis Rosengart and Donna DiGiovanni.

The authors thank Dr. Diana M. Schneider, Publisher, and Joan Wolk, Managing Editor, of Demos Medical Publishing, for assistance in the development and publication of this book.

1

What Is Progressive Multiple Sclerosis?

We assume that you are reading this book because your physician has told you that the multiple sclerosis (MS) you live with is the *progressive* form of the disease, and you want to understand more about the nature of progressive disease and its impact on your life.

Before discussing progressive MS specifically, and because many of you may have been first diagnosed with MS some years ago, we will start with a review of our current understanding of this disease.

Multiple sclerosis is the major neurologic disorder diagnosed in young adults. It affects the *central nervous system* (CNS), which is made up of the brain and spinal cord. The MS disease process produces tiny microscopic lesions of damaged tissue in both areas. The *peripheral nervous system*, which is made up of the many peripheral nerves and muscles, is generally entirely spared. The lesions of MS show a number of characteristic features (Table 1.1). First, there is *inflammation*, in which immune system cells from the blood, such as T cells, B cells, and monocytes, cross the *blood–brain barrier* to move into the brain and spinal cord. This typically occurs right around a blood vessel. This inflammation is often accompanied by localized *edema* (water fluid) as a sign of the temporary marked leakiness of the blood vessels.

Once the blood immune cells are within these CNS tissues, they cause local immune reactions. Immune reactions normally do not occur within the CNS. When they do, they result in *demyelination*. Myelin is

Table 1.1   *Characteristic Features of the Multiple Sclerosis Lesion*

- Inflammation (blood immune cells move into the CNS)
  — Initial/very early feature
- Edema (leakage of water into the CNS)
  — Initial/very early feature
- Demyelination
  — Begins early/more pronounced later feature
- Axon Damage and Loss
  — Begins early/more pronounced later feature
- Oligodendrocyte Loss (glial cell population that makes myelin)
  — Marked loss occurs only in a proportion of patients
  — Patients with marked loss do not remyelinate
- Remyelination
  — Later feature
  — Occurs only in a proportion of patients
- Gliosis
  — Later feature
  — Scarlike reaction of major glial cell population (astrocytes)

made up of lipids (fats) and proteins that form an insulating sheath around the nerve fibers, called axons (Figure 1.1). This insulating myelin sheath allows very rapid electrical nerve impulse conduction. The CNS can be thought of as a computer system that controls the whole body through electrical cross talk (nerve impulses). All the nerve cells of the CNS connect through their axons. Loss of insulating myelin eventually leads to failure of nerve conduction.

One of the surprising recent findings is that a number of people with MS show an impressive amount of myelin repair (*remyelination*). This can occur right next to an area of myelin destruction. However, some MS patients show no remyelination. It has only been appreciated very recently that MS also involves damage to the nerve fibers, or axons. This seems to be particularly important in people with MS who have a progressive course. A scarlike reaction (gliosis) occurs surrounding the damaged area. The actual lesions are called *plaques*; they tend to form most often (but not always) around small blood vessels and very near *cerebrospinal fluid* (CSF), a waterlike liquid that surrounds and cushions the brain and spinal cord. People with MS have dozens to hundreds of plaques of varying ages within their brain and spinal cord. These lesions tend to occur during waves of disease activity and are formed over many years throughout the course of MS. In these lesions the CNS cells that make the myelin sheath, called *oligodendrocytes*, are often destroyed. One oligodendrocyte myelinates many axons (Figure 1.2). In those individuals who show remyelination,

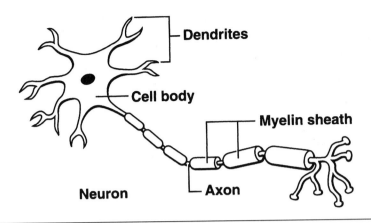

Figure 1.1 *Myelinated Axon*

both precursor cells and surviving cells divide to create new oligodendro-cytes; in those patients who do not remyelinate, there is no replenishment of new oligodendrocytes. One of the progressive forms of MS (primary progressive) seems to be associated with a marked loss of oligodendrocytes and the absence of remyelination.

Who Develops Multiple Sclerosis?

Multiple sclerosis shows a number of unusual features (Table 1.2). It is a disease that affects young people rather than older individuals. Approximately 90 percent of MS patients have onset of their disease between the ages of 15 and 50. It is unusual to have disease start at the extremes of age. Fewer than 1 percent have onset of their disease in childhood (under the age of 10), and fewer than 1 percent have onset of their disease late in life (over the age of 60). Only 2 to 6 percent of patients show signs of MS before age 16. The age of onset of MS can influence the disease course. Progressive MS is more likely to occur in people who develop the disease at an older age.

Multiple sclerosis shows a strong gender preference. Approximately 70 to 75 percent of all people with MS are women. The only exception is a particular form of progressive MS referred to as *primary progressive* MS, which involves men as often as women; patients with this form of MS most often show clinical features that suggest involvement of the spinal cord. This progressive form is discussed further below. The explanation for the female predominance in MS is not clear. However, most autoimmune or

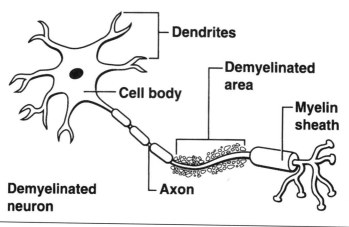

Figure 1.2 *Demyelinated Nerve*

strongly immune-mediated diseases show a female predominance. This may relate to the fact that immune responses in general tend to be stronger in women than in men, perhaps putting them at greater risk for diseases that involve an overactive immune system.

Caucasians account for more than 90 percent of all people with MS. The disease is very rare in Africans and Native Americans. African Americans show a mixed frequency of MS between that of Africans and Caucasians. This may reflect mixing of the gene pool, resulting in an in-between risk of developing the disease. However, they appear to develop more severe MS than Caucasians. Multiple sclerosis is also uncommon in Asians.

How Common Is Multiple Sclerosis?

At least a million people and possibly up to 2.5 million people worldwide have MS. In the United States, estimates have ranged from 250,000 to 350,000 individuals with symptomatic disease. Epidemiologic studies that look at numbers and locations of people who have MS have turned up a number of peculiar findings about the disease. First, MS is not evenly distributed. There are geographic areas that have only a few cases (so-called low-risk zones) of fewer than 5 people per 100,000 population affected. Other areas have a modest number of MS cases (medium-risk zones) of 5 to 30 people with the disease per 100,000 population. Finally, there are regions with a high number of cases (high-risk zones) with greater than 30 individuals per 100,000 population. There are even some "hotbed" areas, such as the Shetland and Orkney Islands off Great Britain, with several

Table 1.2   *Characteristic Clinical Features of Multiple Sclerosis*

- ■ Affects Young Adults
  - — Most newly diagnosed patients range from age 15 to 50 years
  - — The average age of onset is 28–30 years
- ■ Shows Gender Preference
  - — 70–75% of people with MS are women
- ■ Most Common in Caucasians (ca. 90%)
  - — Western European, Scandinavian background
  - — None in Africans, Native Americans
- ■ Variable Clinical Course
  - — Relapsing disease (episodic acute disease attacks/flare-ups)
  - — Progressive disease (gradual worsening)

hundred people with MS per 100,000 population. Most of the studies that have been carried out to map the number of people with MS worldwide have found a very low number living at the equator and a steadily rising number as you move north and south of the equator. For example, MS is much more common in Canada than in the United States, and within the United States it is much more common in the North than in the South.

What Causes Multiple Sclerosis?

The cause of MS is not known for certain, but three factors appear to play a role: the genes we inherit, the environmental exposures we have in life, and our immune system.

Genetics

Only 20 percent of people with MS report a relative who also has the disease. However, there are a few "hotbed" families in which multiple members have developed MS. When a relative has the disease, the risk of MS steadily increases the closer the affected relative. The risk of MS is greatest when a sister or brother has the disease (approximately 3–4%), is next highest when a parent has the disease (approximately 3%; interestingly, the risk is slightly greater when the mother rather than the father is affected), and is 2 to 3 percent for a parent whose child has the disease.

Overall, having a close relative increases your risk of MS 20 to 50 times over the risk for someone without an affected relative. Although this suggests a genetic role for MS, it is clear that MS is not an "inherited" disease. Several groups have searched the entire human genome looking for a critical MS factor. They have been unable to find a gene that causes MS. When a racially homogeneous population of MS patients is studied, however, a number of genes can be identified that are *associated* with increased risk of developing the disease, as well as genes that are associated with more severe or milder disease. These associated risk and severity genes change when one examines a different racial MS population.

To date, no universal disease-associated genes have been found in MS. The genes that are associated with MS all deal with immune system responses and are referred to as *immune response genes*. The simplest way to explain these gene associations is to say that the immune system we inherit is a critical factor for the development of MS. Either one can inherit an immune system that makes it possible to develop MS if there are certain exposures at specific time points in life or one can inherit an immune system that makes it impossible to develop MS, no matter what environmental exposures may occur.

Multiple sclerosis involves more than just genes. Although twin studies find greater *concordance* for MS (shared disease development) between monozygotic (genetically identical) twins than between dizygotic (nonidentical fraternal) twins, the concordance rate of genetically identical twins is no greater than approximately 40 percent. Twin studies indicate that other factors, in addition to the genes we inherit, must play a role in the development of MS. There are rare instances of MS occurring in patients with a defined gene mutation. However, in the vast majority of people with MS gene mutations do not seem to be responsible for the disease. The genetic data on MS can be summarized as indicating that MS is not an inherited disease and cannot be passed on from parents to children. However, we do inherit genes that determine and control our immune system. Genes that affect the immune system appear to convey risk for, or protection against, subsequent development of MS.

Environment

A number of environmental factors have been thought to play a role in MS. Studies have looked at such diverse items as diet, sunlight exposure, and toxin exposure. However, the environmental factors that are most likely to play a role in MS are common infectious agents that we are exposed to—both viruses and bacteria. Perhaps a person who inherits a certain immune system and who is then exposed to environmental infections early in childhood is somehow set up to have his or her immune system later attack the CNS. No single infectious agent has been implicated in MS, and no single virus or bacteria has been consistently isolated from MS tissue. At the current time, a number of pathogens are being studied in MS (Table 1.3). Among the most interesting are a herpesvirus called human herpesvirus type 6 (HHV-6) and a bacterial agent called *Chlamydia pneumoniae*. Both of these are common agents, and many people without MS have been infected with these agents.

The relationship between infection and MS is complicated. It is known, for example, that benign viruses that cause the common cold can trigger MS disease attacks. There is similar evidence, although not as strong, that bacteria that cause urinary tract infections can also precipitate MS disease flare-ups. All people with MS, as compared with 90 to 95 percent of control populations, appear to have antibodies to another herpes virus, the Epstein-Barr virus (EBV). This virus typically causes either infectious mononucleosis or an asymptomatic illness when it first invades the body. Once a herpesvirus, such as EBV or HHV-6, or certain other agents invade the body, they persist for life in a *latent* (hidden) form. One of the difficulties in interpreting the infectious agent data in MS is that we now know that all individuals, even healthy controls, can have latent infectious agents in their CNS tissue. Since MS is a disease that involves both CNS inflammation and abnormalities in the immune system, it might become easy for a latent agent to be reactivated in the CNS and then detected. However, the agent might have no role in why that individual developed MS in the first place.

At the current time, studies are ongoing to determine whether any of the agents listed in Table 1.3 are truly important to MS. It may be that a given infectious agent plays a role only in a subset of individuals and that several agents will ultimately be linked to MS. Alternatively, it could be that environmental pathogens are only of importance from a historical perspective, as a triggering event, and do not actively infect MS patients. Finally, it is possible that these agents have no significant role in MS.

Table 1.3   *Infectious Agents Implicated in Multiple Sclerosis*

Viruses
- Human herpesvirus type 6
- Epstein-Barr virus
- Herpes simplex virus
- Retrovirus
- Canine distemper virus

Bacteria
- *Chlamydia pneumoniae*
- Unidentified spirochete

The Immune System

The final factor implicated in the development of MS is the person's immune system. It is known that blood immune system cells, particularly activated T cells and B cells, will traffic into the CNS. In MS these activated lymphocytes apparently recognize local nervous system antigens and are "turned on" locally. The resultant localized immune response within the CNS leads to damage of CNS tissue and production of the classic MS lesions referred to as plaques.

Very recent studies indicate there may be distinctive immune pathologies in different subgroups of MS. Some people appear to have their CNS immune damage solely mediated by T lymphocytes and macrophages, which are important antigen-presenting cells as well as scavengers of the immune system. Others seem to have CNS immune damage mediated by antibody and a family of soluble proteins called *complement*, which interact with antibody to injure cells. Still other people with MS seem to have a disease process that involves destruction of the glial cells that make myelin in the CNS (oligodendrocytes). These oligodendrocytes appear to be dying as the result of a primary attack that may not involve immune damage.

At the current time, these observations on the diverse pathology of MS are under intense study. If they can be confirmed, it will support the concept that MS is immunologically heterogeneous. This would mean that different immune responses are responsible for CNS damage in subsets of MS. In this case, optimal treatment would need to be tailored, depending on the subgroup of MS.

Clinical Subtypes of Multiple Sclerosis

Multiple sclerosis is variable in severity and is clinically heterogeneous, encompassing a spectrum of severity and clinical patterns (Table 1.4). At the mildest end of the spectrum, MS is "clinically silent." This is referred to as *asymptomatic* or *subclinical* MS. Such individuals have the disease pathologically yet never manifest overt neurologic problems. Such a diagnosis is detected only at autopsy or brain biopsy. Studies indicate that this asymptomatic silent MS may account for 20 to 30 percent of all cases.

When MS declares itself and is clinically diagnosed, the two major patterns are *relapsing* disease and *progressive* disease. They are distinguished strictly by clinical criteria: the time course of onset of neurologic problems. *Relapsing-remitting* MS is characterized by intermittent disease attacks. Patients are clinically stable between attacks (Figure 1.3). Relapsing MS

Table 1.4   *The Clinical Subtypes of Multiple Sclerosis*

Asymptomatic MS
- Based on autopsy studies
- Estimated to make up 20–30% of all MS

Symptomatic MS

Relapsing
- Acute disease attacks; stable between attacks
- 85% of all MS at onset
- Overall accounts for about 55% of MS
- Includes benign (10–20%) subgroup

Primary Progressive
- Slow worsening from onset; never experiences acute attacks
- 10% of MS
- Affects men as often as women

Progressive Relapsing
- Slow worsening from onset; later experiences acute attacks in addition to slow worsening
- 5% of MS
- Very similar to primary progressive subtype

Secondary Progressive
- Relapsing MS patients who later develop slow worsening (90% by 25 years from diagnosis in untreated patients)
- Overall accounts for about 30% of MS
- Patients may continue to have less frequent acute attacks or may stop having attacks altogether

Proposed Classification Revisions
- Combine primary progressive and progressive relapsing
- Divide secondary progressive into with and without relapses
- Combine relapsing MS with incomplete recovery/increasing permanent deficits and secondary progressive MS

---

patients have disease *relapses*, also called attacks, exacerbations, or flare-ups. By definition, relapses involve neurologic problems that occur over a brief period of time—typically days but sometimes as short as hours or even minutes—to mimic stroke in a young adult. These attacks most often involve motor, sensory, visual, or incoordination (cerebellar) problems early in the disease course; bladder, bowel, sexual, and cognitive problems may be seen in later attacks. Sometimes the attack onset occurs over several weeks. The typical MS relapse involves a period of worsening, with development of neurologic deficits, then a plateau period, in which the patient is not getting any better but also not getting any worse, followed by a recovery period. Recovery usually begins within a few weeks.

Types and Courses of MS

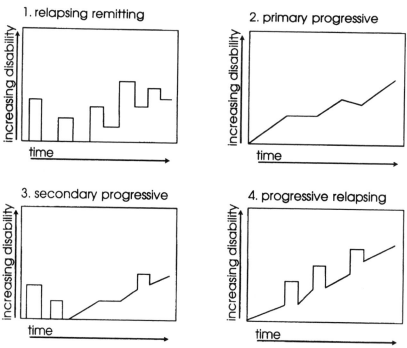

Figure 1.3 *1. Relapsing-remitting (RR) MS is characterized by clearly defined acute attacks with full recovery or with sequelae and residual deficit upon recovery. Periods between disease relapses are characterized by lack of disease progression. 2. Primary progressive (PP) MS is characterized by disease showing progression of disability from onset, without plateaus or remissions or with occasional plateaus and temporary minor improvements . 3. Secondary progressive (SP) MS begins with an initial RR course, followed by progression with or without continuing relapses. 4. Progressive relapsing (PR) MS shows progression from onset with subsequent relapses.*

Recovery from an MS relapse is never guaranteed. People tend to make a complete recovery after their early relapses but incomplete recovery after their later relapses. Most people with MS (85%) start out with the relapsing form of the disease. Among these relapsing patients, a subset show very mild disease, which is referred to as *benign* or mild relapsing MS. These individuals have few MS attacks. The attacks they do experience are very mild, and they show excellent recovery. Their neurologic examination remains virtually normal or minimally abnormal over time. Their disease has little to no impact on their ability to work, and they function normally. Ultimately, benign relapsing MS is a retrospective diagnosis. It requires being able to look back at someone who has had the disease for 25 to 30 years and show that they have minimal associated disability. The best review of the available literature suggests that only 10 percent of people with MS who are followed up longitudinally truly fall into this benign subgroup. A recent epidemiologic study from Northern Ireland is particularly bothersome. In this study, half of the patients who appeared to have benign disease after 10 years had progressive MS and significant disability after 20 years.

A second general form of the disease is referred to as *progressive* MS. People with progressive MS show a gradual development of neurologic deficit independent of relapses. It may literally take months of observation to appreciate that someone is slowly losing function. Three forms (clinical subtypes) of progressive MS have been defined by expert consensus (Table 1.4). Fifteen percent of people with MS start out with a progressive form. They have either *primary progressive* MS (10%) or *progressive relapsing* MS (5%). These patients often start out with difficulty walking because of leg weakness. The third and major progressive subtype is *secondary progressive* MS. People who develop secondary progressive disease start out with relapsing MS. Years into their relapsing course they begin to slowly worsen and basically transition from a relapsing stage to a progressive stage of MS.

As noted previously, most individuals with MS begin with relapsing disease. However, because relapsing patients often convert to progressive disease, when one examines the entire population of MS patients, 55 percent are relapsing, 30 percent are secondary progressive, 10 percent are primary progressive, and 5 percent are progressive relapsing (Table 1.4).

All patients with relapsing MS are at risk for transition to secondary progressive MS. This transition occurs most often in people with relapsing disease who have reached a certain level of disability and who are beginning to have limitations in their ability to walk. At this stage, a relapsing patient is at high risk to transition to progressive disease within a short period of time (a year or two). Other warning signs of transition to progressive MS are an increase in clinical relapses, poor recovery from relapses, and relapses that involve multiple neurologic abnormalities:

- Clinical attacks normally decrease over time so that patients with a longer duration of MS have fewer relapses than patients in the early stages of their disease. Therefore, an increase in the attack rate in relapsing patients who have had MS for several years is a warning sign that they are in danger of entering a secondary progressive stage.
- Early in MS most people show full recovery from their relapses. In MS patients who have had their disease for five or more years, incomplete recovery from relapses—the gradual accumulation of permanent

deficits—is another warning sign that they are at risk for transition to secondary progressive MS.

■ A change in the nature of relapses also indicates the possible onset of progressive MS. In patients who have had MS for five years or more, a relapse that involves multiple neurologic deficits (e.g., motor, sensory, and incoordination) is a warning sign of transition to progressive MS.

Recently, there have been discussions concerning whether the clinical subtype classification should be revised to better reflect current thinking about this disease (Table 1.4). One or more of these changes may be adopted in the next few years.

2

The Diagnosis of Progressive Multiple Sclerosis

Before we can discuss how progressive multiple sclerosis (MS) is diagnosed, we need to first review how the disease is diagnosed when it first appears. Many people reading this book will have had MS for some time, and the diagnostic process has changed substantially in the past 10 to 15 years.

For many people, MS is now a treatable disease, and an early and accurate diagnosis is more important than ever before. Appropriate diagnosis avoids any further and unnecessary diagnostic workups, determines whether a person is eligible for MS disease-modifying therapy, and avoids inappropriate therapies. In addition, accurate diagnosis allows one to predict the likely disease course. It relieves the stress of the unknown, not only for the person with the disease but also for the family. The diagnosis of MS is ultimately what is termed a "clinical diagnosis" because there is no single laboratory test that can *unequivocally* confirm or rule out the diagnosis. Recognizing the importance of a valid diagnosis, and to minimize misdiagnosis, it seems obvious that clinical criteria are best supported by appropriate laboratory testing (Table 2.1).

The clinical diagnostic criteria for MS were outlined by Schumacher in the mid-1960s. These criteria are:

- that MS should begin at an appropriate age (10–50 years);
- that neurologic abnormalities should involve CNS white matter, with motor, sensory, visual, and coordination problems, rather than

13

Table 2.1   *The Diagnosis of Multiple Sclerosis*

Clinical Features
- Appropriate age of onset (10–59)
- CNS white matter disease
- Evidence of lesions disseminated in time and space
- Documentation of abnormal neurologic examination
- Clinical disease pattern shows either acute attacks lasting at least 24–48 hours and spaced at least one month apart (relapsing disease) or slow worsening for at least six months (progressive disease)
- No better explanation exists
- Diagnosis made by a knowledgeable doctor (preferably a neurologist)

Laboratory Criteria
- Blood Work Excludes Other Diagnoses
  — Vitamin B12, vitamin E levels
  — Erythrocyte sedimentation rate
  — C reactive protein
  — Antinuclear antibody
  — Rheumatoid factor
  — Thyroid-stimulating hormone
  — Cortisol
  — Glucose
  — Anti–*Borrelia burgdorferi* antibodies (Lyme disease)
  — RPR (syphilis)
  — Anti–HTLV-1 antibodies (tropical spastic paraparesis—HTLV-1-associated myelopathy)
  — Anti–HIV-1 antibodies (AIDS)
  — Very long chain fatty acids (adrenoleukodystrophy, adrenomyeloneuropathy)
  — Gene studies to exclude Leber's disease, mitochondrial cytopathies
- Neuroimaging
  — Brain MRI with contrast (gadolinium dye)
  — Spinal MRI with contrast
- Cerebrospinal Fluid
  — Oligoclonal bands
  — Intrathecal CNS IgG production
  — Non-MS studies (cell count, protein, glucose, cytology, VDRL, special tests)
- Other Tests
  — Evoked potentials (visual, somatosensory)
  — Central motor conduction
  — Special bladder studies

involving CNS gray matter, with prominent dementia, seizures, and movement disorder problems;

- that there should be evidence of lesions disseminated in time and space;

- that the neurologic examination should show abnormalities;
- that patients should have either a relapsing course, with neurologic attacks lasting at least 24 hours and two attacks spaced at least one month apart, or a slow stepwise progressive course over a minimum of six months;
- that there should be no better explanation; and
- that the diagnosis should be made by a competent clinician, preferably a neurologist.

These clinical criteria were later modified slightly to broaden the age range for disease onset up to 59 years and to recognize that a clinical relapse could involve brief symptoms lasting seconds to minutes if they occurred repetitively over several days to weeks. An example of such a relapse is Lhermitte's sign, which involves an electric shock–like sensation down the back or into the extremities that is triggered by bending the neck.

The diagnosis of MS is important because it identifies that an individual has a treatable disease, it removes his or her uncertainty, it allows informed planning, and it gives an improved sense of well-being because the person finally has an explanation for puzzling neurologic problems.

The laboratory workup for MS generally involves selected blood studies, magnetic resonance imaging (MRI) of the brain, and cerebrospinal fluid (CSF) examination. Formal criteria for the diagnosis of MS have been set up to use in research studies. For a laboratory-supported diagnosis, this requires one of two possible CSF immunologic abnormalities.

Laboratory Workup for Multiple Sclerosis

Blood Studies

In general, blood studies in individuals suspected of having MS are used to rule out other conditions. These conditions include nutritional deficiencies (vitamin B12 deficiency), infections (Lyme disease; retrovirus infection, including AIDS and human T-cell lymphotrophic virus type 1 infection, which cause progressive spinal cord disease that can mimic progressive MS), collagen vascular disease, vasculitis, and endocrine disturbances

Not all of the blood tests listed in Table 2.1 are done in the individual patient being worked up for a possible diagnosis of MS. Appropriate blood work must be guided by the history and physical examination. The foundation for a diagnosis of MS is always built on a thorough history and examination.

Brain Magnetic Resonance Imaging

Brain MRI is very helpful to support a diagnosis of MS. Early in the disease, brain MRI shows suggestive CNS white matter lesions in approximately 65 percent of patients. Ultimately, brain MRI shows lesions in 90 to 95 percent of MS patients. The characteristic findings are multiple asymmetric lesions situated around the ventricles in the white matter. At the current time, there is no way to look at a brain MRI and say unequivocally that the lesions are due to MS. However, there are specific size, shape, number, and location features that increase the likelihood that lesions are due to MS. In fact, expert consensus groups are now in the process of considering criteria for an MRI-based diagnosis of definite MS that could be used for diagnosis at the time of a first attack.

There is a real advantage to doing a contrast (gadolinium) MRI brain study. Contrast enhancement of lesions indicates damage to the blood–brain barrier that has occurred within the prior six weeks and indicates an active MS disease process. Brain MRI becomes less valuable for diagnosis in a person above the age of 50, when vascular and age-related changes start to produce white matter lesions. In fact, it has been recommended that brain MRI not be relied on to make a diagnosis of MS in someone over age 50. In contrast, spinal MRI does not show any vascular or age-related changes, so that intrinsic spinal cord lesions detected on MRI are very useful to support the diagnosis of MS. Unfortunately, spinal cord MRI shows only 10 percent of the lesion activity of MS. It is therefore not routinely done but is reserved for older patients or patients who present with spinal cord symptoms. This is often most likely to be progressive patients.

Cerebrospinal Fluid Studies

Analysis of CSF can be useful to support a diagnosis of MS. Two immune abnormalities in CSF strongly suggest MS. The first is detection of *oligoclonal bands*, a special type of restricted immunoglobulin G (IgG, the major type of antibody produced by the immune system) pattern that must be seen in spinal fluid but not in blood. Early in MS approximately two-thirds of patients will show oligoclonal bands in their CSF. Ultimately, bands are detectable in 90 to 95 percent of those with MS. Although oligoclonal bands in CSF are not specific to MS and can be seen in chronic infections and inflammatory disorders of the CNS, MS is by far the most common disease in which they occur.

The second CSF abnormality that supports a diagnosis of MS is *intrathecal* (within the CNS compartment) IgG antibody production, which means that IgG is present in the spinal fluid compartment at higher levels than would be explained by leakage of serum. In other words, IgG antibody is being produced within the CNS. This does not happen normally and indicates that inflammatory cells have entered the CNS compartment from the blood. This can be measured by a CSF test called the *IgG index*, which is basically a simple ratio of CSF to serum levels of IgG antibody and albumin protein. A 24-hour IgG synthesis rate is another way to measure intrathecal IgG production. This test uses a formula with values plugged in identical to those used to calculate the IgG index.

Ultimately, CSF intrathecal IgG production is present in 70 to 90 percent of MS patients. It is most likely to be absent early in the disease course. This is true for both of the CSF immune disturbances (oligoclonal bands, intrathecal IgG production). Once they become positive, they stay positive. Other useful CSF features are the cell count and protein level, which can suggest a misdiagnosis. A very high CSF cell count (> 50 to 100 white blood cells) or a very high CSF protein level (> 100 mg/dl) are rarely seen in MS and, if present, suggest another diagnosis. Special CSF tests such as cytology, Lyme serology, or VDRL (to rule out syphilis) are helpful to exclude other conditions in the differential diagnosis of MS. The presence of myelin basic protein in the CSF indicates acute tissue damage but is nonspecific and is not a useful diagnostic test for MS.

Other Tests

Blood studies, brain MRI, and CSF are the major laboratory tools to diagnose MS. Additional tests such as evoked potentials/responses are useful in specific cases. These tests look at nerve conduction and brain wave patterns in the optic nerves and visual system, sensory systems in the spinal cord and higher up, and auditory system pathways in the brainstem and cortex. They can document an unexpected subclinical (silent) lesion by slowing of nerve conduction along a visual, auditory, or sensory pathway. A recent consensus paper suggested that visual evoked potentials, followed by somatosensory evoked potentials, particularly of the legs vs. arms were the most helpful evoked potential tests to diagnose MS. Other tests such as special bladder studies can document a neurogenic bladder and provide evidence of another lesion consistent with MS.

The Diagnosis of Progressive Disease

It is not always easy to tell that a person is in a progressive stage of MS. People with relapsing disease may have incomplete recovery from each attack, with accumulating deficit (see Figure 1.3). However, by current criteria they are not considered to have progressive MS as long as they are stable between attacks. In patients who do have progressive disease, the rate of deterioration can be quite variable. Very gradual worsening may take months to years to appreciate. Patients with progressive forms of MS can be clinically stable for up to several years at a time. They occasionally even show mild improvement, although it does not last. In those who have very gradual deterioration, the diagnosis of progressive disease may require up to a year or two of observation. A slowly worsening course has to be observed for at least six months or more to diagnose progressive MS. Research studies suggest that certain blood and urine tests, brain pathology, MRI changes, and immune system measures are more likely to be found in progressive versus relapsing MS. However, no laboratory test at the present time can truly confirm that someone is in a progressive stage.

The diagnosis of progressive MS is based on clinical observation and examination, with documentation of gradual deterioration and loss of neurologic function. It is often the patient who realizes that he or she is slowly getting worse, even before the doctor detects worsening on neurologic examination. The patient may notice that he or she is no longer able to walk as far without needing to rest, is not doing as well at sports, is no longer able to climb the same number of stairs, or is having increasing difficulty with hand and arm function.

The onset of progressive MS is probably the most powerful predictor of disability. Natural history studies that have looked at untreated MS show that almost all individuals (virtually 100%) with progressive disease for 17 to 20 years need an assistive device to ambulate. Financial studies indicate that progressive MS is more costly than relapsing MS. In 1994 dollars, the cost of medical care in the United States was estimated at $10 billion a year. Costs for the average relapsing patient are about $30,000 a year, whereas costs for the average progressive patient are $50,000 a year.

Characteristics of Secondary Progressive Disease

The most common form of progressive MS is called *secondary progressive*. Everyone with secondary progressive disease starts out with relapsing MS. Most people with relapsing MS stay that way through the first few years of the disease. Beginning several years into relapsing disease, some people develop gradual worsening between their disease attacks—they are moving from a relapsing phase of MS to a progressive phase. Over time, this happens to more and more people with relapsing disease. Natural history studies of untreated

MS show that by 25 years after diagnosis close to 90 percent of untreated patients will have moved into a secondary progressive stage of the disease.

It is not always easy to tell that a person with relapsing disease has become secondary progressive. Even though many abnormalities have been associated much more often with secondary progressive MS than with relapsing MS, none of them can confirm this diagnosis (Table 2.2). Features of the disease that often accompany the development of progressive disease include:

- Secondary progressive patients usually have limitations in their ability to walk. It has been noted that relapsing patients with a Kurtzke Expanded Disability Status Scale (EDSS) in the 4–5.5 range (which is determined by the ability to walk 500 meters or less without rest) tend to worsen and go on to progressive MS within a relatively short period of time.
- They show more abnormalities and disability on neurologic examination compared with relapsing patients. Most secondary progressive patients have an EDSS of 6 or higher (maximum 10) compared with relapsing patients, who typically have an EDSS of less than 4 (higher EDSS indicates a worse neurologic examination).
- Progressive disease is the MS subtype with the highest rate of cognitive problems. Cognitive problems in MS have been related to MRI changes, including an increased burden of disease.

Table 2.2 *Characteristic Features of Secondary Progressive Multiple Sclerosis That Differ from Relapsing Disease*

Patients Have
- Longer duration of MS
- Fewer or no disease relapses
- More abnormalities on neurologic examination
- More prominent cognitive disturbances
- More damage on brain MRI
  - Larger total lesion volume
  - More lesions around the ventricles
  - More confluent (overlapping) lesions
  - More lesions affecting the brainstem, cerebellum, and spinal cord
  - More "black hole" lesions
- An increase in total brain lesion volume that no longer mirrors the number of new contrast enhancing lesions
- More damage to axons, with more brain and spinal cord atrophy
- More pronounced immune disturbances
  - Immune cells produce increased amounts of damaging proinflammatory cytokines
  - Immune cells show less ability to suppress immune responses
  - Blood lymphocytes that attack myelin cannot be inhibited

- Many secondary progressive patients will have very infrequent relapses and ultimately stop having relapses altogether. In fact, one can divide people with secondary progressive MS into those with and those without superimposed relapses.

- Progressive patients generally have more evidence of damage on brain MRI than relapsing patients. This is not surprising because they typically have had MS for a longer period of time. It also explains why they are more likely to have cognitive problems.

- Secondary progressive patients are more likely to have a large volume of lesions in the white matter surrounding the *ventricles*, the inner chambers of the brain that are filled with CSF. Although this anatomic localization of lesions on brain MRI would be consistent with secondary progressive MS, this alone does not necessarily *prove* the existence of this clinical subtype.

- Progressive patients are more likely to have lesions in the back part of the brain, referred to as the *posterior fossa*. This area includes the cerebellum and brainstem. Lesions in these areas can produce problems such as tremor, incoordination, diplopia (double vision), and eye movement disturbances.

- Progressive patients also are more likely to have spinal cord lesions. Lesions in this area often produce problems such as leg weakness, impaired walking, and bladder, bowel, and sexual difficulties.

- One of the most consistent differences between relapsing and secondary progressive MS is that those with progressive disease show more damage to the axon nerve fibers, with actual destruction of axons and measurable atrophy of brain and spinal cord. These axon changes have been shown in pathology studies that directly examine the tissues, as well as on a special MRI technique called MR spectroscopy, which measures chemicals in the brain. One such chemical is called N-acetyl-aspartate (NAA). In the adult brain NAA is found only in axons and neurons. Secondary progressive MS patients show a decrease in whole brain NAA compared with those who have relapsing disease. They also show decreases in NAA in normal-appearing brain tissue. People with secondary progressive disease show more brain and spinal cord atrophy than those with relapsing disease, as measured on MRI. Using another measure of focal tissue loss, secondary progressive MS patients show more "black holes" (areas of brain with destroyed tissue), as measured on T1-weighted MRI (Figure 2.1).

It has been suggested that MRI lesions are more likely to overlap and become confluent in people with secondary progressive disease. In relaps-

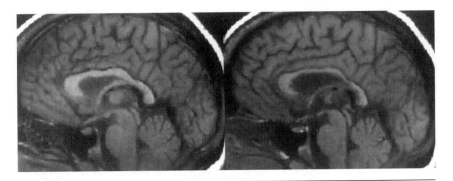

Figure 2.1 *Brain atrophy in multiple sclerosis. On the left, a baseline scan shows a near-normal corpus callosum, a highly myelinated area that connects the left and right cerebral hemispheres. On the right, the same area two years later shows considerable shrinkage due to loss of myelin.*

ing MS, MRI contrast lesion activity appears to correlate with the increasing total *burden of disease* in the brain, a measure of the absolute volume of brain tissue that is damaged. In secondary progressive MS, this correlation is much poorer, and the increasing burden of disease does not necessarily reflect new contrast lesion activity. In fact, certain treatments have been able to stop the development of gadolinium-enhancing lesions in the brain of secondary progressive patients, yet they continue to worsen clinically with an increasing brain lesion burden. This suggests that the lesion burden in secondary progressive MS may be increasing as a result of prior occult damage that cannot be compensated for over time and ultimately produces irreversible permanent CNS damage. Alternatively, patients may lose a protective factor or may enter a stage of their disease in which the major damaging CNS mechanism has changed.

Some very interesting but limited studies have looked at immune disturbances in people with secondary progressive MS versus relapsing MS. Although differences have been reported, these findings are preliminary and need to be studied more extensively. Progressive MS patients seem to produce more *proinflammatory cytokines*. Cytokines are soluble hormones of the immune system. They are very important regulators of the immune response. Proinflammatory cytokines enhance inflammation and worsen the MS disease process. Therefore, any increase in proinflammatory cytokines would be expected to worsen MS. Most people with MS have blood lymphocytes that are reactive (sensitized) to CNS myelin. When these self-reactive lymphocytes are isolated from progressive MS patients, they cannot be shut off in the test tube. In other words, they have lost the ability to be inhibited. In contrast, the same type of damaging lymphocyte, when isolated from relapsing patients, *can* be turned off. Suppressor cell activity, which would be expected to inhibit the abnormal immune responses in MS, is low in MS patients compared with controls. Those with secondary progressive disease show much less suppressor activity than those with relapsing disease. These and other immunologic features could help explain why relapsing and progressive MS show different disease courses. Alternatively, they may reflect changes associated with disease duration or severity. Central nervous system pathology associated with secondary progressive MS has suggested less inflammatory disease, more acute axon injury, and more B cell and macrophage activation than T cell activation.

Characteristics of Primary Progressive and Progressive Relapsing Disease

Primary progressive MS occurs in only 10 percent of patients. This progressive subtype is characterized by a number of specific features (Table 2.3). Many people believe that primary progressive MS is the form of the disease that is most biologically different from the other MS subtypes. By definition, people with primary progressive disease must never have an acute relapse. They tend to have an older age of onset—they are generally older than age 35 and are often in their forties or fifties when diagnosed. The clinical presentation seen in at least 60 percent of these patients is that of a slowly worsening spinal cord syndrome (referred to as a *progressive myelopathy*). They often note a gradual onset of walking difficulty, which becomes noticeable over months to a year or more. Primary progressive disease is the only clinical form of MS that shows an equal sex ratio, with men as likely to be affected as women.

People with primary progressive disease typically show a low burden of disease on brain MRI. They often show little in the way of gadolinium contrast-enhancing lesion activity, and sometimes the brain MRI is even normal. In contrast, the spinal cord seems to bear the brunt of the disease process. It often shows atrophy, with loss of tissue and tissue thinning. This atrophy may reflect in large part the loss of axon nerve fibers. With regard to CNS pathology, primary progressive MS shows less inflammatory change, more axon and oligodendrocyte cell loss, more chronic low-grade axon injury, more microglial cell activation, and less macrophage activation. However, these differences are quantitative rather than qualitative.

Table 2.3 *Characteristic Features of Primary Progressive Multiple Sclerosis*

- Older age onset of disease (typically past age 35)
- Equal gender ratio
- Prominent spinal cord involvement—gradual onset of difficulty walking and prominent spinal cord atrophy
- Brain MRI shows relatively less damage (primary progressive and progressive relapsing) and contrast lesion development as opposed to relapsing and secondary progressive MS

The diagnosis of primary progressive MS requires only that a person has had slow worsening and has never experienced a clinical relapse. It is determined strictly on clinical criteria. The primary progressive form of MS also includes a group of individuals who have a progressive cerebellar syndrome and generally show very disabling tremor and imbalance. Unlike the primary progressive patients with spinal cord disease, those with cerebellar disease may have a very abnormal brain MRI. In fact, the brain MRI looks more like that of a patient with secondary progressive MS.

Although both types of patients are currently considered to have primary progressive MS, it would seem as if they do not have identical forms of the disease. This area is under study. It is important to determine whether there are any true biologic differences from the rest of MS. These differences could be used to diagnose primary progressive disease and might ultimately be useful clues to treat patients. Certainly the fact that most patients show an older age of onset, no female predominance, and spinal cord involvement rather than brain involvement suggests that there are important distinctions from general MS. A group of European experts recently proposed new diagnostic criteria for primary progressive MS that require both clinical and laboratory abnormalities (Table 2.4). These criteria are being tested to see how reliably they identify this type of progressive patient and whether they should be widely accepted.

Progressive relapsing MS is a relatively new classification and is the most unusual form of MS, accounting for only approximately 5 percent of all patients. Progressive relapsing patients show a slowly progressive disease from onset. Early on, they are indistinguishable from primary progressive patients. However, they subsequently experience acute MS attacks. By our current definition, people with primary progressive MS must never have clinical relapses. If they do, they are then reclassified as having progressive relapsing MS. Recent studies suggest that primary progressive and progressive relapsing MS are so similar that it may make more sense to consider them as a single subtype.

Table 2.4   *Proposed Criteria for the Diagnosis of Definite Primary Progressive Multiple Sclerosis*

- Age 25 to 65
- Slow worsening observed for a minimum of one year
- Abnormal CSF (oligoclonal bands or elevated IgG index)
- Positive MRI as determined by
  — 9 brain lesions
  or
  — 2 spinal cord lesions
  or
  — 4 to eight 8 lesions and 2 spinal cord lesions

Identifying Relapsing Patients at Risk for Progressive Disease

Certain characteristics may define people with relapsing MS who are at high risk (in the immediate future) for transition to secondary progressive disease. As a group, relapsing MS patients tend not to have a lot of abnormalities on neurologic examination. This probably reflects in large part that most early MS patients are relapsing and that disease attacks are most often reversible, at least early on. The CNS seems to be able to compensate and recover. As disease duration increases so do neurologic abnormalities, and the neurologic examination becomes more and more abnormal. The CNS can no longer compensate for the MS damage. These patients go on to a secondary progressive phase of the disease.

Relapsing patients with numerous deficits on neurologic examination should be considered at risk for secondary progressive MS. The number of clinical attacks is also a helpful warning sign. The natural history of MS attacks is to decrease over time. Therefore, if the relapse rate is increasing several years into MS, this indicates accelerating disease with greater risk for secondary progressive MS.

Although people with relapsing MS can become secondary progressive at any time, the transition generally occurs 5 to 20 years into the disease. The risk for entering a progressive stage of MS is based somewhat on the age of onset. In those who develop relapsing MS at a young age, progressive disease tends to occur only after a number of years. In contrast, it often occurs much sooner in people who develop relapsing MS at an older age. Some studies suggest that men with relapsing MS are at greater risk for secondary progressive disease than women.

Other warnings signs are a relapsing MS patient who is no longer responding to steroids when he or she has an attack or who is showing a poor response to the "A, B, C" drugs (Avonex®, Betaseron®, and Copaxone®) (see Chapter 3). These relapsing MS patients are becoming refractory to standard treatments. This can be viewed as moving on to a more severe stage of the disease, in which the CNS can no longer compensate for injury. Alternatively, the disease process itself may become more severe. The nature of the last MS attack and the degree of recovery are also helpful warning signs. When attacks involve multiple neurologic abnormalities, such as combinations of motor, bladder, bowel, and sensory disturbances, as opposed to a single abnormality such as vision loss, and when there is incomplete recovery from the last attack in MS, someone who has had relapsing MS for five or more years may be at risk to transition to secondary progressive disease.

As reviewed previously, recent studies suggest MRI differences between relapsing MS and secondary progressive MS. Progressive patients show more axon damage, more brain and spinal cord atrophy, a greater total lesion burden of disease, more "black hole" lesions (which show a less intense signal than surrounding brain), and enlargement of the CSF-filled ventricles within the brain. Therefore, relapsing patients who are developing MRI changes that look like secondary progressive disease may well be announcing that they are moving into a progressive stage of MS.

Gadolinium-enhancing brain lesion activity tends to decrease in the later stages of relapsing MS as patients are moving into the progressive disease stage. Despite this reduction in new lesions, there is an increasing brain burden of disease. As noted earlier, this may reflect prior injury, with eventual loss of cells and axons over time.

CLAYTON-LIBERTY TWP LIBRARY
Clayton, IN 46118

3

Disease-Modifying Therapy

$\mathcal{P}$rogressive multiple sclerosis (MS) appears to involve more axon damage than relapsing MS, with less in the way of inflammatory disease. Therefore, therapies that are anti-inflammatory and are designed to regulate the immune system may not be as effective as strategies designed to protect, or even regenerate, axons and enhance remyelination. The emphasis on treatment of progressive MS is relatively recent. In the first few years of development of MS disease-modifying therapies, there was a focus on relapsing MS, the major subtype. Now that several treatments for relapsing MS are available, there is a new emphasis on the more severe and difficult progressive forms of MS.

Current Treatments for Relapsing Multiple Sclerosis

At the time of this writing, five disease-modifying therapies have been shown to decrease MS disease activity and damage in major multicenter, blinded, placebo-controlled (phase III) trials (Table 3.1). These drugs have worked in relapsing MS to decrease the number and severity of clinical attacks, sustained worsening on neurologic examination, and silent lesion activity on brain magnetic resonance imaging (MRI). In addition, two of the drugs (interferon β-1b/Betaseron® and mitoxantrone/Novantrone®) each showed benefit for secondary progressive MS in a phase III trial.

Table 3.1   *Multiple Sclerosis Disease-Modifying Therapies*

- Cytokine strategy
  Interferon β-1b (Betaseron®)
  Interferon β-1a (Avonex®, Rebif®)
- T cell strategy
  Glatiramer acetate (Copaxone®)
- Immunosuppression
  Mitoxantrone (Novantrone®)

The National Multiple Sclerosis Society has recommended that patients with definite relapsing MS be treated as soon as possible after diagnosis. This recommendation was recently reinforced by a similar endorsement from the Canadian MS Clinics Network, which recommended the treatment of active relapsing patient who are still able to walk.

All the current disease-modifying therapies affect the immune system, but they do so in different ways.

Interferon Beta

Interferon beta is a *cytokine*. As mentioned in Chapter 2, cytokines are hormones of the immune system that are very important regulators of the immune response. Interferon beta, also referred to as a *type 1 interferon* (a category that also includes interferon alpha), is an anti-inflammatory or regulatory cytokine. It opposes or antagonizes proinflammatory cytokines, such as interferon gamma and tumor necrosis factor, which make MS worse. Interferon beta decreases the migration of immune and/or inflammatory cells into the central nervous system (CNS), inhibits lymphocyte activation, blocks the expression of cell surface molecules that would enhance immune responses, increases suppression of cell activity, and stabilizes the blood–brain barrier. Interferon beta also has antiviral and anticancer properties.

The three interferon betas now available to treat MS have been shown in large phase III studies to benefit relapsing MS. They are given at different doses subcutaneously (just under the skin) or intramuscularly. Interferon β-1b (Betaseron®) is given at a dose of 8 million international units (IU) (250 mcg) subcutaneously every other day. Interferon β-1a (Avonex®) is given at a dose of 6 or 9 million IU (30 mcg; the value differs based on the standard used in the assay to measure activity) intramuscularly once a week. Interferon β-1a (Rebif®, not yet available in the United States) is given at a dose of 6 (22 mcg) or 12 (44 mcg) million IU subcutaneously three times a week.

Glatiramer Acetate

Glatiramer acetate, or Copaxone®, is not a cytokine. Rather, it is a *substitute antigen* (also considered an *altered peptide ligand*). Glatiramer acetate mimics myelin basic protein (MBP), a very important component of the CNS myelin sheath and a major immune target in a number of people with MS. Glatiramer acetate consists of random polymers of four amino acids. It is given at a dose of 20 mg subcutaneously daily. The mechanism of action of glatiramer acetate is believed to involve the production of activated anti-inflammatory (suppressor) lymphocytes. These activated lymphocytes preferentially enter the CNS, where they are restimulated locally to produce anti-inflammatory cytokines. These CNS cytokines suppress immune responses that are occurring in the neighboring tissues. Glatiramer acetate appears to inhibit the CNS immune reactions that occur in people with MS through a "bystander" suppression mechanism. These are the local reactions that are responsible for tissue damage and the production of MS plaques.

Thus, glatiramer acetate acts within the CNS, while interferon beta acts outside the CNS. Unlike the interferon betas, which show benefit on MRI parameters within a few weeks and on clinical parameters by three months, glatiramer acetate appears to take longer (2–6 months) to show its full clinical and MRI benefits. This may reflect that it takes some time to generate a large enough population of anti-inflammatory T cells.

Mitoxantrone

Mitoxantrone (Novantrone®) is a cancer drug. It is *cytotoxic* (it interferes with DNA structure and repair in any dividing cell of the body) and is a very strong immune system suppressant. It decreases levels of white blood cells and tends to suppress immune responses, although it does increase suppressor cell activity. Mitoxantrone is given intravenously every three months at a dose of 12 mg per meter squared of body surface, a dose that is carefully monitored because of concerns about cardiac toxicity. There is a limit to how much mitoxantrone can be given before there is an unacceptable risk for heart damage; a dose of 12 mg per meter squared can only be used for three years. In cancer patients who receive higher doses, approximately 2.5 percent develop cardiac (left ventricular function) impairment.

Lower doses (5 mg per meter^2) also have efficacy, and it has been suggested that mitoxantrone could be used for a longer period of time by starting out with the high dose and then switching to the low dose once MS disease activity was controlled. Mitoxantrone is very well tolerated. It can produce nausea, hair thinning, menstrual irregularities, and low white blood cell count. It also can make patients more susceptible to infection. Mitoxantrone in solution is blue and produces a temporary harmless discoloration of body fluids, including urine, tears, and sweat.

Treatments for Progressive Multiple Sclerosis

It is not surprising that optimal treatments for progressive MS might be different from those for relapsing MS. The relapsing stage of this disease is characterized by prominent inflammation, less axon loss and atrophy, less permanent damage, and more potentially reversible CNS injury. The progressive stage has less inflammation, more axon loss and atrophy, more permanent damage, and less potentially reversible injury. It is not necessarily true that a drug that works for relapsing patients will also work for progressive patients. It thus becomes necessary to conduct formal studies to document that a proposed treatment truly works in progressive patients.

A number of treatments are now being tried in people with progressive MS. There are three completed major trials that evaluated interferon β therapy; only one was positive. This was the European study of interferon β-1b (Betaseron®), which involved 718 secondary progressive MS patients who ranged in age from 18 to 55, with an Expanded Disability Status Scale (EDSS) score of 3.0 to 6.5. An EDSS of 3.0 means that there is no limitation in the ability to walk but that there are several detectable abnormalities on neurologic examination; an EDSS of 6.5 means that the individual requires either a walker or bilateral assistive devices to walk any distance.

This secondary progressive MS trial was designed as a three-year study with two arms—interferon β-1b given at the same dose used for relapsing MS (8 million IU subcutaneously every other day) and a placebo treatment. Although the study had been designed to last three years, there was a built-in two-year prospective interim (halfway through) analysis. At this interim analysis, the drug had shown such a clear-cut benefit over placebo treatment that the study was stopped after two years. The placebo recipients were then offered the drug. The primary outcome was time to confirmed progression.

Interferon β-1b treatment, as compared with placebo treatment, slowed time to confirmed progression by 11.5 months during the two-year study period. This was highly statistically significant. Among the secondary endpoints, in the 70 percent of patients who continued to have relapses, interferon β-1b treatment decreased relapses by 31 percent. This was also statistically significant compared with the placebo-treated patients. With regard to MRI disease parameters, at the end of two years the placebo-treated patients had an 11.9 percent increase in brain burden of disease. In contrast, the interferon β-1b–treated group had a 5.2 percent reduction in total brain burden disease. This also was a statistically significant difference. Interferon β-1b treatment decreased active lesions on brain MRI by 65 percent in the first six months of the study and by 78 percent in the final six months of the study. Interferon β-1b decreased the proportion of active scans by 29 percent in the first six months of the study and by 49 percent in the last six months.

Patients in this study were a more severe group of patients than typical relapsing MS patients, yet they tolerated interferon β-1b therapy very well. Depression was carefully looked for, and patients who were actively depressed or suicidal were screened out. No increase in depression was found during the study. Spasticity is one of the side effects that is more common when interferon beta is used to treat more severely affected progressive patients. Spasticity was increased in the treated group and occurred in 38 percent of patients compared with 27 percent of placebo-treated patients. Except for this one feature, the side effects of interferon beta were no different in progressive MS compared with relapsing MS.

The major side effects were flulike reactions and injection-site reactions. These adverse effects were rarely bothersome enough to stop treatment. Flulike reactions to interferon beta can be minimized when starting therapy by three steps: (1) giving the dose during early evening; (2) starting at a low dose and increasing to full strength over the next few weeks; and (3) premedication with anti-inflammatory drugs during the first few weeks of therapy. Giving interferon beta in the evening means the drug peaks during sleep, 6 to 10 hours later. There are various dose escalation schedules, which typically start at 25 percent or 50 percent dose for the first two weeks and then escalate as tolerated to full dose. During the first few weeks of therapy, premedication should be done consistently, using ibuprofen (Motrin®), acetaminophen (Tylenol®), naproxen (Aleve®), pentoxyphylline (Trental®), or other medications. Ibuprofen three times a day for the first several weeks was shown in a small controlled trial to be very effective, along with dose escalation, in reducing flulike side effects. Injection site reactions are minimized by use of an automatic injection device, good technique, appropriate selection of injection sites, use of a small clean needle, and injection of room temperature drug.

The European study using interferon β-1b for secondary progressive MS showed very positive benefits on both clinical and MRI disease parameters. Unfortunately, the later North American study of interferon β-1b for secondary progressive MS did not confirm an effect on slowing disease progression. Treatment did benefit other clinical measures (particularly relapses) as well as MRI disease measures. This means that the European and North American trials gave opposite results.

A careful comparison of both studies suggests that this different result is best explained by the fact that the studies involved slightly different populations of secondary progressive patients. The European secondary progressive patients were at an earlier stage of their disease, with continued relapses and contrast CNS lesion activity. The North American patients were later in the secondary progressive stage of disease, with limited relapses and contrast lesion activity.

These two studies teach us something important about secondary progressive MS. To see the most benefit from an agent such as interferon beta, it probably is critical to treat early and particularly to treat progressive patients who are still having relapses and an inflammatory disease component. The interferon betas are effective primarily against the inflammatory component of MS. It is likely that different treatments will be needed to manage axon damage and loss, which appears to be primarily responsible for increasing disability in people with progressive disease. It was only about 30 percent higher than the fixed dose.

The North American study had a third arm based on body size (5 MIU/m^2). This dose was chosen to try to minimize side effects, but it did not show any benefit over fixed-dose treatment.

Other trials have looked at other interferon betas in secondary progressive MS. There was a three-year study of interferon β-1a (Rebif®) (the SPECTRIMS trial) conducted in Europe and Canada. This was also a negative study because there was no significant effect on the primary outcome (an effect on sustained progression). A very puzzling feature was a gender-based treatment effect. Interferon β-1a treatment worked for women with secondary progressive MS but not for men with secondary progressive MS. Similar to the North American interferon β-1b study, many other disease parameters (clinical attack rate, need to use steroids, MRI parameters such as new lesion development and total burden of disease) were all statistically significantly better in the interferon β-1a (Rebif®)–treated patients compared with placebo-treated patients. There was also a dose-response curve, with the higher dose giving better results than the lower dose. If certain pretreatment factors were controlled for (neurologic exam, duration of disease, rate of worsening), the primary outcome—sustained progression—became statistically significant in favor of interferon β-1a treatment. In addition, in secondary progressive patients who had experienced relapses in the two years before the study, interferon β-1a treatment had a positive effect on progression time that almost reached statistical significance. It was interesting that the secondary progressive patients without relapses who entered the SPECTRIMS trial were significantly older, had a longer disease duration, and had been in the progressive phase of their MS for a longer period than the secondary progressive patients with relapses.

The North American study of interferon β-1a (Avonex®) for secondary progressive MS is close to completion. This study is using double-dose interferon beta-1a (Avonex®), 60 mcg intramuscularly once a week. It is a two-arm study, with placebo and interferon beta treatment groups. The primary outcome does not involve EDSS changes but rather a composite of three tests to evaluate timed walk, hand function, and mental processing speed.

A small pilot study of interferon β-1a (Avonex®) for people with primary progressive disease, which evaluated both 30 and 60 mcg doses, recently reported a modest benefit on one MRI parameter in favor of the 30 mcg treatment. No other outcome measure was affected. The significance of this limited benefit is unclear, and further studies in primary progressive MS are warranted.

Glatiramer Acetate

A major trial of glatiramer acetate for primary progressive MS is now under way. The PROMISE trial involves more than 50 centers in North America and Europe and includes over 900 people with primary progressive MS. One-third are receiving placebo, while the other two-thirds are receiving subcutaneous daily injections of glatiramer acetate.

The rationale for testing glatiramer acetate in primary progressive MS is based on earlier work. A chronic progressive study of glatiramer acetate was carried out in the early 1980s at two centers (Albert Einstein in New York, New York, and Baylor Medical Center in Houston, Texas) that included individuals with both primary and secondary progressive MS. Although the overall results were negative, glatiramer acetate was successful at the Einstein center. In a retrospective review of patients who would qualify as primary progressive, there was a trend toward benefit from glatiramer acetate. The PROMISE trial should provide a definitive answer as to whether glatiramer acetate treatment benefits primary progressive MS. It should also provide a great deal of important information on clinical, MRI, and laboratory aspects of this unusual progressive subtype. At the current time, it is not known whether glatiramer acetate therapy benefits secondary progressive MS.

Immunosuppression

A number of immunosuppressant strategies have been tried for progressive forms of MS (Table 3.2). The only one supported by a major (phase III)

Table 3.2   *Immunosuppressive Therapy of Progressive MS*

■ Mitoxantrone (Novantrone®)
■ Azathioprine (Imuran®)
■ Methotrexate
■ Cyclophosphamide
■ Cladribine (Leustatin®)
■ Total lymphoid irradiation
■ Bone marrow transplantation

trial is mitoxantrone (Novantrone®), which is now approved by the U.S. Food and Drug Administration (FDA) for use in worsening (relapsing and secondary progressive) MS. At this time it is the only approved drug for secondary progressive disease in the United States. The trial was conducted in relapsing and secondary progressive MS patients in Europe and Canada and awaits publication. Presented data indicate that during a two-year study the drug showed benefit over placebo treatment, based on both clinical and MRI disease parameters. Mitoxantrone is a cytotoxic cancer drug that interferes with DNA and DNA repair mechanisms. It attacks dividing cells, including immune system cells.

Patients in the two-year study ranged in age from 18 to 55, with EDSS scores of 3.0 to 6.0. A patient with an EDSS of 3.0 can walk without difficulty but has abnormalities on neurologic examination, whereas a patient with an EDSS of 6.0 requires a cane to walk any distance. The study involved three treatment arms: placebo, low-dose mitoxantrone at 5 mg per meter^2 of body surface, and high-dose mitoxantrone at 12 mg per meter^2. Treatments were given by intravenous infusion over 5 to 15 minutes every three months for two years.

Patients who received mitoxantrone benefited on multiple clinical parameters. The EDSS, the overall neurologic rating scale, was significantly lessened in both treatment groups compared with the placebo group, where the EDSS increased at the end of two years. Other significantly improved outcomes included a positive effect on the ambulation index (walking ability) in favor of high-dose mitoxantrone; a decrease in the average number of relapses in both mitoxantrone treatment arms; a significant delay in the time to first treated relapse in the high-dose treatment group; a significant decrease in patients with confirmed six-month disease deterioration with high-dose mitoxantrone (7% vs. 19% in the placebo group); a significantly higher percentage of patients who did not require treatment for relapses (72% with high-dose mitoxantrone vs. 44% with placebo); and a positive treatment effect on the average number of relapses and time to first relapse.

In addition to these clinical parameters, there was a positive effect on MRI disease parameters. Contrast-enhancing lesions were effectively shut off. This was more marked at two years than at one year, particularly with high-dose mitoxantrone. In addition, both treated groups showed a reduction in new lesion formation, with the most impressive decrease in the high-dose group. This trial, along with prior studies, led the FDA to approve mitoxantrone for relapsing and secondary progressive MS. A small pilot study is now evaluating mitoxantrone therapy in primary progressive MS.

Mitoxantrone is well tolerated. The most common side effects are nausea, hair thinning, menstrual abnormalities, leukopenia (lowered white blood cell count), and increased risk of infection. There are rare cases of late leukemia in patients who received mitoxantrone and other chemotherapeutic agents as well as radiation therapy. However, the risk of this drug appears small in patients with good cardiac status and no extensive history of irradiation or other immunosuppressive agents.

A number of other forms of immunosuppression have been used to treat progressive MS. All remain unproven, although initial reports are promising for bone marrow transplantation. These include:

- Azathioprine (Imuran®) is usually taken orally in doses of 50 mg to 300 mg daily to lower the white blood cell count below normal range. Studies with azathioprine have not shown overwhelming benefit. The drug has a slow onset of action and takes months before it is fully effective.

- Methotrexate is an orally administered agent that is generally taken once a week at doses that range from 7.5 to 20 mg. This drug is widely used to treat rheumatoid arthritis, systemic lupus erythematosus, and psoriasis. In one study, it was shown to slow loss of hand and arm function in progressive MS patients compared with placebo. However, this slowing of progression did not seem to make a significant functional difference.

- Cyclophosphamide (Cytoxan®) can be given orally or, more commonly, intravenously. This drug has the potentially significant side effect of long-term bladder cancer. It is excreted in the urine and requires that patients be well-hydrated to avoid injury to bladder tissue resulting in blood in the urine. Patients being treated with cyclophosphamide have an increased risk of infection, hair loss, and infertility. Cyclophosphamide generally is used for aggressive MS. However, it is not as well tolerated as mitoxantrone.

- Cladribine (Leustatin®) is given by subcutaneous infusion. In initial studies, this drug seemed to stabilize progressive MS patients.

Unfortunately, patients worsened quickly once the drug was stopped and within a year looked no different from placebo-treated patients. In a more recent multicenter phase III trial in primary and secondary progressive patients, cladribine did not slow disease progression. This drug is no longer being used for MS.

- Total lymphoid irradiation was reported to show a benefit in progressive MS. The treatment had to lower the white blood cell count in order to work. This treatment produces permanent changes in body tissues; it subjects the body to significant radiation for very modest benefit and has not been pursued as an MS treatment.

- Bone marrow transplantation can be used to replace an abnormal immune system. Patients undergo intensive immunosuppression and radiation to destroy their current immune system and then have their own immune system reconstituted by infusion of stem cells (immature cells taken from the patient's own bone marrow and blood that develop into adult immune system cells). At the current time, *autologous* stem cell transplants are being used, in which the cells are harvested from the MS patients themselves before they undergo intensive immunosuppression. This approach has been chosen because the mortality rate is relatively low (3–8%). However, better results may be obtained from *allogeneic* transplants, in which stem cells are harvested from a closely matched but healthy donor. At the current time, this allogeneic approach is limited by an unacceptably high mortality rate of 15 to 30 percent. However, new techniques may bring this mortality rate down close to the autologous rate. If this could be accomplished, healthy stem cells rather than MS stem cells would be preferred to decrease the risk of disease relapse after several years. Although bone marrow transplantation appears to be promising for progressive MS, it remains unproven. It is costly (about $100,000), carries a small risk of death, does not improve fixed deficits, and in preliminary studies has only been demonstrated to stabilize patients for one to two years. It is not known whether it works for prolonged periods or whether prolonged benefit will require allogeneic stem cells versus the currently used autologous stem cells.

Other Therapies

Other therapies that have been used to treat progressive forms of MS include pulse intravenous high-dose glucocorticoids. Typically, intravenous methylprednisolone (SoluMedrol®) is used, given as a 1 gram infusion over 30 to 60 minutes one day a month. No major trials have shown this treatment to be beneficial, but anecdotal evidence suggests that some progressive patients may improve for a period of time. Intravenous immunoglobulin (IVIG) infusions have also been used to treat progressive MS, but there is no standardized protocol. Typically, IVIG is infused over several hours, one or two days each month or every other month. Ongoing studies are evaluating the efficacy of this treatment for progressive MS.

Central Nervous System Repair Strategies

There is great interest in CNS repair strategies as future treatment for progressive MS. These techniques would repair fixed damage, at least in major lesions that are responsible for significant clinical problems such as leg weakness, imbalance, or vision loss. The goal of this therapeutic approach is to enhance remyelinization, protect axons, and promote axon regeneration. Central nervous system repair strategies offer the hope that function can be restored and fixed deficits can be improved.

By definition, progressive MS patients have fixed deficits that are increasing. They are the optimal candidates for CNS repair strategies. At the current time, there are a number of potential ways to boost CNS repair (Table 3.3). Although preliminary studies are beginning in MS patients, most repair strategies are being developed in animal models. They include cell transplantation to produce remyelination, treatment with trophic factors to cause axon sprouting and regrowth and division of precursor cells to form new myelin-making oligodendrocyte cells, and immune manipulation to promote myelin repair. Intravenous immunoglobulin therapy has been helpful to promote remyelination in animal models, although two recent human studies failed. A recent animal model study found that a specific immunoglobulin promoted remyelination, and this monoclonal antibody is being evaluated for use in MS patients. There also is the possibility of using gene transfer techniques to promote axon recovery, remyelination, and survival of both myelin-making cells and axons.

Table 3.3 *CNS Repair Strategies*

- Cell transplantation
- Growth factor therapy
- Immune manipulation
- Gene transfer
- Neuroprotection

These CNS repair strategies will need to be combined with a disease-modifying treatment for the ongoing disease process. They probably will be targeted to specific lesions because most MS plaques are clinically silent (i.e., they produce no detectable symptoms on neurologic examination). Prime targets for remyelination and axon regeneration would be, for example, a critical lesion in the spinal cord that has caused a paralysis of both legs causing an inability to walk or a critical lesion of the optic nerve that has caused permanent and significant vision loss; in such cases, the goal would be to restore or improve the lost function.

Other CNS repair strategies include *neuroprotective* strategies aimed at the neuron and its axon processes. It is only very recently that CNS repair strategies—including the emphasis on axon protection, axon repair, and axon regeneration—have been stressed as a treatment approach to MS. This reflects our better understanding of the MS damage and disease process and the critical importance of axon involvement to explain permanent MS deficits. Axon damage is particularly prominent in progressive MS.

Combination Therapies

Future treatment of MS is likely to involve combination drugs, very similar to the manner in which cancer is treated. This will be necessary until we are truly able to cure or prevent MS. A number of studies are evaluating various combination therapies. In a pilot study, approximately 30 MS patients were treated with a combination of interferon β-1a (Avonex®) and glatiramer acetate (Copaxone®). These two disease-modifying therapies act on different parts of the immune system. Although they may be additive or synergistic (helpful to each other), there has been some concern that they could interfere with each other's benefit. Interferon beta blocks cell migration into the CNS, while glatiramer acetate requires cell migration of activated anti-inflammatory cells into the CNS in order to work. Therefore, this combination could interfere with and block each other's benefit. In the pilot combination study, patients were monitored to make sure that when the drugs were added together they did not result in an increase in brain MRI lesions. No increase in disease activity was noted, so the combination therapy appeared quite safe. Improved efficacy needs to be established.

In addition to the combination of interferon beta and glatiramer acetate, investigators are looking at "adding on" immunosuppressive agents, either as a preliminary step to take control of the MS disease process and optimize the subsequent response to treatment or as an add-on agent to ongoing disease-modifying therapy to improve the therapeutic response. These combination strategy treatments include oral azathioprine, methotrexate, or cyclophosphamide and intravenous mitoxantrone or cyclophosphamide. Pulse glucocorticoids or IVIG are also being studied. There are a number of other potential combination drug treatments using a second agent to enhance the response to disease-modifying therapy. In the next few years, we are likely to see many combination therapies being tested in MS, including progressive patients. Axon-protective or axon-restorative agents would seem to be particularly valuable to use in people with progressive MS.

4

Managing the Symptoms of Progressive Multiple Sclerosis

In its early stages, multiple sclerosis (MS) generally produces mild and intermittent symptoms that can usually be managed by medical and self-care intervention. Each attack (exacerbation, flare-up) and each new symptom or change in function requires that a person readjust to a changing situation. The goal of managing MS is to assist the person with the disease and his or her family and friends to make room for this ever-changing condition without giving it more space, time, or energy than it absolutely needs.

When MS becomes progressive, symptoms that previously were episodic often become persistent. At this stage, they are more likely to affect quality of life. These changes may be subtle at first, only to increase in intensity and duration to the point that they alter daily activities. It is extremely important to identify those symptoms that have such a negative impact and to seek treatment to reduce and control them. It may be helpful to make a list of your symptoms in rank order of how bothersome they are and their importance. This list can be brought along and discussed during your doctor visits. Managing these symptoms may involve lifestyle changes, physical management, the judicious use of medications, and possibly surgical options.

Although each person's disease pattern varies a great deal from its onset and from day to day, symptoms, functional problems, and psychosocial concerns are very common in MS. This chapter seeks to help those of you coping with the ongoing challenges of MS through symptomatic management.

41

Fatigue

Fatigue may be the single most disabling symptom of MS in people with progressive disease. Fatigue superimposed on other problems can have a very negative effect on daily activities. Fatigue is defined as an overwhelming sense of tiredness, lack of energy, or feeling of exhaustion. This feeling of exhaustion in healthy individuals often accompanies mild "flu-like" illness. However, the fatigue of MS is quite different from what healthy people experience. It often comes on without warning and does not require an exertion trigger. It is distinct from depression (lack of self-esteem, despair, feelings of hopelessness) as well as from motor and/or muscle weakness.

Fatigue can be chronic and severe or intermittent. It can predate a relapse, accompany one later, or come on independently. It can occur at any stage of the disease and may occur in patients with almost normal examinations. Up to 90 percent of people with MS experience fatigue problems. One of the unique features of MS fatigue is that is is temperature-sensitive: heat, particularly humid heat, typically makes fatigues worse, while cooling can improve fatigue. Sensitivity to heat is typical of a number of other MS symptoms as well, but it is not a feature shared by people with fatigue resulting from other chronic diseases.

New onset of fatigue may be the initial signal of another problem. It may be the sign of an impending relapse, it may signal a urinary tract infection (UTI) or some other infection, or it may represent depression masquerading as fatigue. People with MS also report tiredness resulting from activities such as using a wheelchair, moving about, and working. Some medications may cause fatigue, including some that are used to treat spasticity such as baclofen or tizanidine. MS fatigue does not correlate highly with age or neurologic impairment. It spans all levels of MS neurologic disability and disease classifications.

Despite the minimal relationship between physical activity and fatigue, physical activity probably relates to at least some aspects of fatigue. People with MS who participate in physical activity can become more fatigued, particularly in a very hot environment. MS fatigue has been associated with impaired motor functioning so that the person must strain to lift, walk, or maintain sitting balance.

There are some reports of sleep disturbances in MS, which may have been missed as a common cause of fatigue. However, sleep problems do not fully explain this very difficult symptom. Abnormalities of sleep such as nocturnal *myoclonus* (muscle movement or night spasms); sleep apnea, in which a person stops breathing periodically; periodic leg movement; and poor sleep efficiency may occur in MS. Your physician should rule out these abnormalities as possible contributing factors to fatigue.

Some cognitive effects of fatigue have been noted. When fatigued, people with MS have prolonged reaction times compared with those who are less fatigued. Fatigue can also affect tests of complex attention to sustained cognitive effort. On the other hand, treating fatigue has very little effect on most of the cognitive deficits associated with MS (see below).

There is no one proven universal cause of MS fatigue. The mechanism underlying this problem has been proposed to include immune dysfunction (production of cytokines and other immune activation factors), central conduction defects, peripheral muscle problems, medications, disturbed sleep, and psychological factors. The physician may also consider preexisting psychological vulnerability to fatigue with illness because some people have a history of becoming fatigued when they are ill. People directly benefit from the fact that their symptoms are recognized as genuine. Although medical conditions are rarely significant factors, thyroid disease, anemia, or other conditions may occasionally be a contributing factor and must be considered.

Coping with Fatigue

Managing fatigue requires a multidisciplinary approach encompassing various factors that might contribute, such as mood, level of physical activity, pain, medication use, and sleep hygiene (Table 4.1). Nonpharmacologic treatments may include education, support, and rehabilitation.

Exercise is a powerful way to combat deconditioning and enhance self-esteem. A graded exercise program may be very useful to treat fatigue. At the same time, overexertion can be limiting as the body becomes overheated. Exercise can be combined with proactive cooling techniques, including cold drinks, proper clothing, rest periods, air-conditioning, and cooling devices. Rest periods during the workday and avoidance of environmental factors that worsen fatigue have also proven to be beneficial. Such environmental factors may include hot meals and drinks and a smoky, poorly ventilated workplace.

Behavior modification is also important in helping people cope and restructure their daily lives to minimize fatigue and produce what is called *effective energy expenditure*. Nonpharmacologic activities such as rehabilitation, rest, and exercise often can be supplemented with medications. One commonly used medication is amantadine hydrochloride (Symmetrel®). This antiviral agent has been shown in several studies to be beneficial in

Table 4.1 *Management of Fatigue*

- Review history and examination for evidence of nonneurologic conditions
  — Thyroid disease
  — Anemia
  — Infection
  — Malignancy
- Review sleep habits
  — Correct any problems to ensure good sleep hygiene
- Review current drugs
  — Discontinue or replace fatigue-inducing medications
- Schedule rest periods/early afternoon nap
- Assess daily activities for energy-conserving techniques
- Institute proactive cooling techniques
  — Frequent cold drinks
  — Air-conditioning
  — Light clothing
  — Cooling devices
- Institute regular aerobic exercise program
  — Three times a week for 40 minutes
- Medications
  — Amantadine (Symmetrel®)
  — Modafinil (Provigil®)
  — Methylphenidate (Ritalin®)
  — Amphetamine mixed salts (Adderall®)
  — Fluoxetine (Prozac®)
  — Pemoline (Cylert®)
  — Amphetamines
  — Caffeine

managing and reducing MS fatigue. Based on the relative benefit of amantadine and its very low side-effect profile, it is considered to be the first-line medication for use in MS fatigue.

If no benefit is obtained from amantadine, the next option is increasingly modafinil (Provigil®), an agent approved for narcolepsy (a sleep disorder characterized by excessive daytime sleepiness). Another option is pemoline (Cylert®), a central nervous system (CNS) stimulant. Pemoline in high doses may result in liver problems, so your physician will need to monitor liver enzyme blood tests while you are taking this medication. Other medications that have been reported as beneficial are antidepressants such as fluoxetine (Prozac®) and CNS stimulants such as amphetamine mixed salts (Adderall®) or methylphenidate (Ritalin®). Caffeine also may improve fatigue.

In a study examining the long-term efficacy and safety of 4-aminopyridine (4-AP), a chemical compound that may improve nerve conduction in MS, fatigue was frequently reported as improved. This treatment is not U.S. Food and Drug Administration–regulated and is under investigation in a sustained-release form.

Improved sleep hygiene is important for people whose fatigue is associated with a sleep disorder. Exercise six hours before sleep may be helpful. Medications for insomnia also may lower fatigue in selected people. Fatigue occasionally may be associated with anxiety or panic attacks. Alleviating these symptoms with appropriate therapies may be beneficial in such cases. Fatigue is a multifaceted problem and is common in neurologic disorders, particularly MS. For many people it is their primary complaint. Interest in this difficult symptom has grown in recent years and should lead to much improvement in its evaluation and management.

Spasticity

Spasticity is an increase in muscle tone that occurs when muscles are stretched (e.g., during exercise, in transfers, or by remaining in one position for a prolonged period). It is a common symptom in people with progressive MS and often is due to spinal cord damage. Spasticity may be so severe as to make it impossible to bend a joint or move the legs apart. Uncontrolled *flexor* (bending) responses involve the legs bending in response to a stretch. *Extensor spasms* involve stiffening of a limb, with an inability to bend the joint. Spasticity may be triggered by a full bowel or bladder, a UTI, or an infected bed sore. These problems that heighten spasticity are called *noxious stimuli*. Hypertonia or spasticity is always accompanied by impaired voluntary movement.

Spasticity can have different effects on people with MS. Mild spasticity may impair ability to walk, make it harder to walk, or limit the distance that can be walked. Severe spasticity may occur in more disabled people who become quadriplegic or paraplegic, causing problems with sitting or transferring. Painful spasms may occur, particularly when sitting or lying in one position for prolonged periods. Untreated spasticity can result in fibrous *contractures*, which permanently bend and limit movement of the joints at the arms, legs, or shoulders.

Spasticity is a very treatable symptom; many treatments are available for this disabling and uncomfortable problem, which can impact all activities of daily living (Table 4.2). All current medications act at different levels of the spinal cord. Major and well-established treatments for spasticity include baclofen (Lioresal®), tizanidine (Zanaflex®), diazepam (Valium®), clonazepam (Klonopin®), gabapentin (Neurontin®), and dantrolene

Table 4.2 *Management of Spasticity*

- Identify and treat any triggering factors
  — Infection
  — Relapse
  — Positioning
  — Skin breakdown
- Institute regular stretching and exercise programs
  — Heat or cold applications to loosen muscles
- Start oral first-line medications
  — Baclofen (Lioresal®)
  — Tizanidine (Zanaflex®)
  — Combination
- Use oral second-line medications as needed
  — Benzodiazepines, such as diazepam (Valium®) and clonazepam (Klonopin®)
  — Gabapentin (Neurontin®)
  — Dantrolene (Dantrium®)
  — Others
- Consider nonoral and/or surgical options
  — Baclofen pump
  — Botulinum toxin A (Botox®) injections
  — Ablative surgery (rarely needed)

(Dantrium®). Baclofen is the most commonly used medication at doses ranging from 5 mg to as high as 120–180 mg a day. This medication reduces both muscle stiffness and the frequency and intensity of acute spasms.

One of the side effects of baclofen is muscle weakness, so it is advisable to start at a very lose dose and increase the drug slowly (titrate it up) until maximal benefit is reached. The goal is to reduce spasticity while maintaining function and without becoming too weak. *The sudden and abrupt withdrawal of baclofen can cause seizures and confusion; if you have been taking this medication for a long time, you must decrease it very slowly if you desire to stop.*

Other medications to reduce spasticity include tizanidine (Zanaflex®), which is available in 2-mg and 4-mg tablets that can be taken in doses up to 36 mg a day. Tizanidine is particularly good for nighttime spasms. Side effects include fatigue, decreased blood pressure, and altered control of urination. It is important to discuss your bladder management with your doctor and/or nurse before using tizanidine in order to avoid problems with incontinence. Because baclofen and tizanidine act at different sites in the nervous system, combination therapy may work better than either drug alone. When combined, each is used at a lower dose than when only a single drug is used. Diazepam (Valium®) and clonazepam (Klonopin®) are both members of the benzodiazepine family. They have a sedative effect (causing sleepiness) and carry the risk of becoming habit-forming. Gabapentin (Neurontin®) can also help spasticity, but it has not been as widely studied as baclofen or tizanidine. Dantrolene (Dantrium®) has been used predominantly for people with spinal cord injury. It acts directly on the muscle. Those who are taking this medication must be carefully monitored for their liver function. Botulinum toxin (Botox®) can be injected into a muscle and will partially paralyze that muscle for up to three months. It may be a helpful therapy when spasticity is limited to specific large muscles.

Baclofen can now be administered *intrathecally* (delivered directly into the spinal fluid through a small catheter that is threaded into the spinal canal). The catheter is connected to a computerized pump that is placed surgically under the skin, usually on the left side of the abdomen. The pump is about the size of a hockey puck and may be programmed to deliver up to 10 different doses of baclofen over 24 hours. A very low dose will be effective compared with when the drug is taken orally. This surgical procedure is usually reserved for people who have had a poor response to oral therapy. The effect of intrathecal baclofen is long-lasting, with benefit for both spasticity and quality of life. The frequency of refilling the pump's reservoir varies with each person based on the severity of spasticity and the dose required to sustain benefit. The pump must be replaced every few years.

For those people who are unresponsive to oral antispasticity agents, the use of the pump facilitates personal care by reducing spasticity in the lower extremities. Bowel and bladder function may improve as a result of decreased tone of voluntary muscles (bladder and anal sphincter). Pain reduction is also a potential benefit if pain is due to muscle spasms. Although side effects of intrathecal baclofen are less than those of the oral preparations, they can include alterations in bowel and bladder patterns (particularly incontinence); changes in mental status (confusion or lethargy), especially if the person is put in a position in which the head is lower than the rest of the body; and potential weakness of the lower extremities if too much medication is delivered by the pump.

Spasticity can also be reduced through regular stretching, proper positioning in bed (side-lying with supports for the back and legs), regular stretching and range of motion exercises, aquatherapy, in which the joints are put through range of motion under water, and a structured physical therapy (PT) program prescribed by a physician. Intermittent PT for spasticity has proven to be very effective not only for teaching the person with

MS new strategies but also in releasing tightened muscles that have been shortened from prolonged sitting and immobility.

Tremor

Tremor is one of the most puzzling and disabling symptoms in MS. In contrast to spasticity, which is hypertonia or increased muscle tone, tremor reflects ongoing muscle movement and may result in involuntary shaking of the head, arms, body, or legs except during sleep. Tremor probably is the most difficult symptom of MS to treat and is one of the most disabling in terms of interfering with performance of daily activities.

A person may have very good strength yet still be unable to perform any voluntary movements because of the intensity of the tremor. Tremor produces a risk of dropping things and inflicting self-injury when trying to use a fork or spoon and may make simple tasks such as buttoning clothing, operating a computer, or writing virtually impossible.

Action tremor is the most common type of tremor in MS. Another name for it is *intention tremor* because it occurs when one tries to *do* something—eat, dial a telephone, or open a door with a key. The movement is completely incapacitating for some people. Others may have only minor problems that minimally interfere with activities. This occurrence of tremor is usually independent of any exacerbation and is due to a secondary degenerative process that disrupts control of voluntary movement, generally in pathways in the brainstem and cerebellum.

Other types of tremor are less common. They include *resting tremor* and *postural tremor*, which occurs during sustained posturing such as outstretching arms. Tremors tend to disappear during sleep.

Attempts to treat tremor usually are disappointing. Many different drugs have been tried with only poor results; a management approach to tremor is outlined in Table 4.3. Propranolol (Inderal®) and isoniazid (Isotamine®) have been of some interest, but there have been only anecdotal reports of benefit. Primidone (Mysoline®), clonazepam (Klonopin®), carbamazepine (Tegretol®), and valproate (Depakote®) have also been tried. The major problem with most treatments for tremor is that they tend to be sedating, making the patient sleepy and at risk for falls. Some newer anticonvulsants, gabapentin (Neurontin®) and lamotrigine (Lamictal®), may possibly be useful, but studies with these agents are limited. There have been anecdotal reports of expensive tremor reduction using ondansetron (Zofran®), an antinausea medication, but a recent placebo-controlled study was negative.

Table 4.3   *Management of Tremor*

- Identify type of tremor, body parts involved, any triggering factors
- Optimal use of assistive devices
  — Therapy evaluation to identify helpful devices
  — Institute use of devices (may include such items as neck or back braces/supports, weighted wrist guards and utensils)
- Medication
  — Propranolol (Inderal®), mysoline (Primidone®), clonazepam (Klonopin®)
  — Gabapentin (Neurontin®), lamotrigine (Lamictal®), carbamazepine (Tegretol®), phenytoin (Dilantin®)
  — Isoniazid (Isotamine®)
  — Ondansetron (Zofran®)
- Surgery
  — Stereotactic neurostimulation
  — Stereotactic neuroablation

The difficulty in managing tremor is that *palliative* treatments (treatments that ease or reduce symptoms without curing the disease) are seldom successful. In the majority of cases, the use of an effective drug results in side effects that are out of proportion to potential effectiveness. For example, clonazepam (Klonopin®) is widely used with some reports of benefit. However, this drug can produce sedation.

The fact that no striking pharmacologic breakthrough has occurred in tremor suggests that strategies from the rehabilitation field should be investigated; these may be beneficial in the future. Rehabilitation measures such as attaching light weights to the wrists and using neck and back supports may be helpful. However, formal outcome studies have not documented functional improvement. To date, nothing has reduced or eliminated tremor.

Surgical procedures to treat tremor have involved both neuroablation (creating a permanent lesion) and neurostimulation (implanting wires—electrodes—that can be turned on or off to stimulate specific brain areas). These procedures have been used mainly for Parkinson's disease and essential tremor, but preliminary reports suggest that thalamic stimulation may benefit MS patients with tremor.

Future approaches may include robotic arms and the use of pulsed magnetic fields to the brain.

Pain

One of the myths in MS is that pain is not a major symptom of the disease. This myth can be particularly demoralizing and emotionally draining for those experiencing this hard-to-tolerate yet invisible symptom. Those around the person with MS may also have a difficult time understanding how disabling this symptom can be. In fact, pain is just another form of a (positive) sensory disturbance caused by the disease.

It is important that anyone experiencing pain consider the possibility of a non-MS cause or explanation. These possibilities include dental problems causing facial pain, arthritis resulting in joint pain and low back pain, and generalized, nonspecific discomfort resulting from poorly fitting wheelchairs, orthotics, or other assistive devices. However, pain is a common feature of MS and affects a high percentage of those with the disease. It can be a primary symptom directly associated with the disease itself or a secondary symptom resulting from inadequate management of a primary symptom. Table 4.4 summarizes common causes of pain in MS and their management.

Pain can be a direct result of demyelination of pain pathways in the brain and spinal cord, or it can be a consequence of damage induced by the disease. For example, pain can result from poorly managed spasticity; sitting for prolonged periods on an uncomfortable cushion in either a wheelchair or a regular chair; or poor posture while ambulating and not using the proper assistive devices (canes, crutches, walker). The therapeutic approach in these cases should involve optimal positioning and improvement in posture, application of ice or moist heat (low setting) to tender muscles, massage, or PT.

Table 4.4   *Management of Pain*

- Identify and treat precipitating factors
  - Spasticity/contractures
  - Poor posture
  - Vascular headaches
- Acute pain medications
  - Carbamazepine (Tegretol®), phenytoin (Dilantin®)
  - Nonsteroidal anti-inflammatory agents
- Chronic pain medications
  - Tricyclic antidepressants (amitriptyline—Elavil®, nortriptyline—Pamelor®, imipramine—Tofranil®), gabapentin (Neurontin®)
- Physical techniques
  - Hot/cold compresses
  - Acupuncture
  - Trigger point injections
- Surgery
  - Facet blocks

Approximately 40 to 50 percent of people with MS complain of chronic pain, and another 30 to 35 percent will experience some pain during their disease course. Less frequently, pain can be of a *paroxysmal* nature (intermittent and stabbing), such as trigeminal neuralgia (see subsequent section). Pain is more frequently experienced by people with more advanced disease and those who are older. In a person with a relapsing disease course, pain may be associated with sensory attacks that result in numbness, tingling, or a binding sensation. These symptoms may last several weeks to several months after the acute phase and may lead to depression and anxiety over the ongoing problem. Treatment should be initiated promptly to avoid the emotional toll of such sustained symptoms.

Pain in MS is classified into three categories: acute, paroxysmal, or chronic. Central neurogenic pain is a direct result of MS. It is caused by demyelination in the CNS sensory tracts. These pathways control transmission and regulation of painful stimuli. MS-related pain can be differentiated from other types of pain by some of its clinical characteristics. People with MS describe it as grinding, gnawing, or burning. It usually is located in the trunk or in a particular area of the body. Some people even describe this type of pain as severe hypersensitivity, a feeling that they do not want to be touched because the skin on the affected body part or parts is exquisitely sensitive.

Trigeminal Neuralgia

Trigeminal neuralgia is probably the most characteristic acute pain associated with MS; it affects 1 to 2 percent of people with the disease. It occasionally occurs on both sides of the face (bilateral), but it is more common on only one side of the face (unilateral). It is due to a plaque, with demyelination or scarring of the fifth cranial nerve. It is very important to recognize trigeminal neuralgia and to differentiate it from facial pain caused by dental caries or periodontal disease. Some people with MS have undergone multiple tooth extractions before the diagnosis of trigeminal neuralgia was finally made.

The treatment of trigeminal neuralgia is aimed at reducing abnormal firing along the fifth cranial nerve. Carbamazepine (Tegretol®) is frequently used to treat this condition. This drug can be effective in higher doses, but sometimes the side effects (lethargy, mental cloudiness) can become intolerable. The most frequently reported side effect is fatigue, which also can be extremely disabling. Other medications used to manage trigeminal neuralgia include phenytoin (Dilantin®), clonazepam (Klonopin®), baclofen (Lioresal®), gabapentin (Neurontin®), amitriptyline (Elavil®), and opiate analgesics. A recent European study found that amitriptyline was more effective in managing dysesthetic pain than carbamazepine (Tegretol®). If trigeminal neuralgia is due to an exacerbation of MS, treatment with intravenous steroids may be helpful.

Some people with MS complain of chronic neuralgia, with frequent attacks during the course of the disease. Misoprostol (Cytotec®), a long-acting prostaglandin-E analogue (prostaglandins are thought to influence nerve transmission; an analogue is a product that is similar to the original) has been found to be safe and may be effective either alone or in combination with other drugs.

Surgical intervention may be required if the pain becomes persistent and disabling and does not respond to management with oral medications. Such surgery may be noninvasive (without actually entering the body), invasive (entering the body), or chemical. It involves destroying the nerve cells and adjacent root, either permanently or temporarily. Temporary chemical destruction of the nerve may be accomplished with an injection of glycerol into the affected area. Radiofrequency thermal rhizotomy (interruption of the nerve) can be effective and may eliminate the need for high doses of oral medications. This noninvasive pain reduction strategy uses external beam radiation to deaden the affected nerves, and its benefits may last for weeks to several months. This procedure is performed by a neurosurgeon and usually is only recommended when all other measures have been unsuccessful. It may need to be repeated.

Other Painful Symptoms

Other painful symptoms such as tonic seizures or Lhermitte's sign (shooting pain down the back or the arms when the neck is bent) are generally relieved by antiseizure drugs such as carbamazepine (Tegretol®), gabapentin (Neurontin®), or clonazepam (Klonopin®) or by the antidepressant amitriptyline. Subacute pain (nagging, gnawing, or aching pain) can be a warning sign for a problem such as a UTI, infected bed sore (decubitus), poorly managed spasticity, poor sitting posture, problems with balance, or ill-fitting assistive devices, such as braces, on the lower extremities.

Pain in the legs can be a manifestation of chronic MS pain. People may complain of burning in the feet of legs and occasionally in the arms and the trunk. This may be associated with discoloration or mottling of the skin. This type of pain is difficult to manage, but elevating the legs or applying cool compresses (or even icing) may be of benefit. Physical therapy (stretching, range of motion) to relieve muscle cramping and improve circulation may be helpful. Compression hose (support stockings or TEDS®) may reduce discoloration by improving blood flow to the legs. Nonsteroidal anti-inflammatory drugs (ibuprofen) may also be beneficial. Painful leg spasms or cramping are part of a more general problem with spasticity that is discussed later in this chapter.

Bladder Dysfunction

Urinary symptoms affect 75 to 90 percent of people with MS over the course of the disease. Difficulty with bladder control is as common a problem as impaired mobility, and these two problems often go hand in hand because they both are often the result of spinal cord disease. The nerves that supply both the bladder and the genitalia originate in the lower part of the spinal cord. Therefore, demyelinating disease in the spinal cord means that the nerves to both the legs and the bladder are likely to be affected. Clinically, bladder control may deteriorate at the same time as leg weakness and spasticity worsen. This makes it increasingly difficult to toilet oneself, clean oneself, and perform other types of hygienically necessary functions.

Bladder dysfunction in MS causes many symptoms. People with MS may experience more frequent UTIs (Table 4.5) or skin breakdown resulting from incontinence. They also may report a poor urinary stream, double-voiding (in which two separate attempts are needed to complete urination), hesitancy when they get to the bathroom, and an inability to void without straining or sitting for a while. The management of bladder dysfunction is directed at treating and reducing symptoms and improving quality of life. The first step in treating bladder dysfunction is to identify the problem.

Table 4.5   *Symptoms of Bladder Infection*

- Fever and chills
- Urgency
- Frequency
- Incontinence
- Nocturia
- Double-voiding
- Change in urine odor or color
- Burning on urination
- Pain in the lower back or flanks

Types of Bladder Dysfunction

Two syndromes may occur in MS, either singly or together. One is called *failure to store*, in which the bladder stores only a small amount of urine from the kidneys before it goes into spasm. The person has to urinate very frequently, emptying fully, but is unable to store urine for prolonged periods. This type of problem results in the need to remain close to a bathroom at all times, with frequent bouts of incontinence.

The other syndrome is called *failure to empty*, in which the bladder muscle becomes weak and is unable to empty fully. Therefore, the person has greater risk of UTIs from urine that is stored for long periods of time. This problem may also result in incontinence, wetting oneself due to overflowing urine along with a feeling of incomplete emptying.

To further complicate matters, a third syndrome may occur, a problem called *bladder-sphincter dyssynergia*. When this syndrome occurs, the large muscle of the bladder—the *detrusor*—may contract to empty the bladder; at the same time the *sphincter*, the muscle at the neck of the bladder, squeezes shut rather than relaxing as it should. These two muscles thus act in opposition to one another. Symptoms of this problem include urgency, frequency, hesitancy, incontinence, nocturia, and UTI.

In addition, the pressure created within the bladder as the two muscles work in opposition to one another can cause urine to reflux (back up) into the kidneys, thus creating the risk of *hydronephrosis* (water-logged kidneys) as a result of "wrong way" flow of urine.

Treatment

Treatment depends on the type of bladder problem you have (Table 4.6). The first thing to check is to make sure that there is no UTI. This can be assessed by a dipstick (which changes color if there are substances present in the urine consistent with infection) or a urinalysis (in which urine is examined under the microscope to detect white blood cells and bacteria). If necessary, a urine culture and sensitivity can be performed. You should suspect an infection if you notice a change in urine odor or color, burning on urination, or pain in the lower back or flanks. Once an infection is ruled out, the next step is to determine whether there is a failure to store, a failure to empty, or a dyssynergic bladder. Symptoms generally will suggest which one is present. It is very important to do a *postvoid residual* to determine the volume of urine left in the bladder after urination, which should be less than 100 ml ($3\frac{1}{3}$ ounces). This can be done by means of a bladder

Table 4.6   *Management of Bladder Problems*

- Diagnose and treat any urinary tract infection
  — Maintain sufficient fluid intake
  — Vitamin C
  — Cranberry juice
  — Appropriate antibiotics
- Determine which type of neurogenic bladder is present (based on symptoms, postvoid residual from bladder scan or catheterization, urodynamics)
  — Failure to store (spastic
  — Failure to empty (flaccid)
  — Disconnected (detrusor-sphincter dyssynergia)
- Spastic bladder
  — Regularly timed urination
  — Anticholinergic medication (oxybutynin—Ditropan®, Ditropan XL®, propantheline—Pro-Banthine®, dicyclomine—Bentyl®)
  — Antimuscarinic medication (tolterodine—Detrol®)
  — Scheduled fluid intakes
  — Scheduled/prompted urination
  — Avoid/minimize bladder irritants (alcohol, aspartame, caffeine)
- Flaccid bladder
  — Intermittent catheterization
- Disconnected bladder
  — Anticholinergics/antimuscarinics
  — Intermittent catheterization
  — Antispasticity agents

ultrasound, in which the instrument is held over the lower abdomen and gives a volume readout in less than a minute. An alternative method is to catheterize the patient and measure the volume of urine removed.

Patients with a spastic bladder have a normal postvoid residual. Patients with a large postvoid residual and dribbling incontinence have a flaccid (failure to store) bladder. In this case, the treatment of choice is to learn how to pass a catheter into the bladder on a regular basis to empty it. This can be thought of as "physical therapy" for the bladder.

The combination bladder (sphincter dyssynergia), which has difficulty voiding, may be associated with either a normal postvoid residual or an increased postvoid residual. It often needs to be treated with medications to relax the bladder along with a catheterization program to empty it. Antispasticity agents may be used to relax the sphincter muscle.

If a person cannot manage to self-catheterize, a member of the family, a care partner, or an attendant may be enlisted to help with this procedure. As one catheterizes regularly, a more normal urinary pattern may become established. If that occurs, the frequency of catheterizations may be reduced. In a few extreme cases in which no assistance is available, an *indwelling* (Foley) catheter may be placed permanently to empty urine from the bladder. Because urine must not remain in the bladder for long periods of time (there is a high risk of infection, which may even be life-threatening), catheterization is the only option when other bladder-emptying methods are not possible.

The person with a bladder that fails to store urine can be treated with medications to reduce bladder spasms and prolong storage of urine. The treatment of choice is a class of medications called *anticholinergics*. Side effects are dry mouth and constipation, and people with glaucoma or uncontrolled high blood pressure may not be able to take these medications. Drugs in this class include oxybutynin (Ditropan® and Ditropan XL®—a new sustained-released product), propantheline (Pro-Banthine®), and dicyclomine (Bentyl®). A new class of drug, an antimuscarinic, tolterodine (Detrol®) relaxes the large muscle of the bladder, the detrusor. This medication is available in 1-mg or 2-mg tablets and has also been found to be beneficial for urinary urgency, frequency, and incontinence. Side effects include dry mouth, headache, and constipation.

Other strategies to improve bladder function include following a high acid/ash diet to acidify the urine (increased white meats and fish and reduced red meats, plus decreased amounts of green vegetables such as broccoli, milk and milk products, and citrus fruits), avoiding caffeine and caffeine products, drinking adequate amounts of fluid, maintaining a regular voiding schedule of every 3 to 3.5 hours, and promoting regular bowel elimination. A full bowel stimulates the bladder and can increase and promote bladder dysfunction. In addition, research has found that untreated constipation can lead to UTIs because of the large bulk of stool remaining in the pelvic area. Regular evacuation patterns are desirable goals for both bowel and bladder function. Cranberry juice and cranberry tablets may reduce the risk of UTI by reducing the urine bacterial count.

Aerobic training has been reported to enhance wellness and fitness in MS. Bladder function improves indirectly with fitness training. Reducing bladder symptoms is essential in the management of MS. Any type of infection can temporarily worsen the disease, so prevention of UTIs will improve quality of life for those affected by MS.

Bowel Dysfunction

Bowel problems are common in MS. Approximately 53 percent of people with the disease complain of constipation, while a smaller number complain of bowel urgency, involuntary bowel movements, or diarrhea. The basis for bowel symptoms is less clear than for the bladder. The central role of the spinal cord in bowel function is well known, and in MS it is primarily spinal cord involvement. However, spinal cord involvement is not the only explanation for bowel dysfunction.

A number of factors may contribute to bowel symptoms, including insufficient fluid intake or fiber in the diet, immobility, slow movement of fecal material, spasticity, and diminished sensation around the perineal area. The clinical features of bowel problems include constipation, diarrhea, fecal incontinence, and, as mentioned earlier, involuntary bowel. People with more advanced disability have difficulty starting bowel movements because of muscle weakness and the use of medications that slow the transit of stool through the intestine.

Managing the elimination of solid waste takes time. A bowel management program may take weeks to months before it is maximally effective. General measures include sufficient fluid intake, a well-balanced diet with adequate fiber, the use of stool softeners and bulking agents, and establishing a regular time for evacuation (Table 4.7). Bladder and bowel problems often go together. Restricting fluids in order to decrease urination, which is often done by patients, not only is potentially harmful to bladder status by increasing the risk for infection, but also will contribute to constipation. Suppositories, mini-enemas, and digital stimulation have been reported to improve bowel function and restore regular bowel movements. It also is important to understand that a daily bowel movement is not always necessary. The regular pattern that one established before the onset of MS should be the goal; this may involve bowel movements every day, every other day, or every third day. However, it is important not to go more than every three days without a bowel movement; fecal material tends to dry out in the intestine as water in the stool is reabsorbed by the gut, causing it to become more difficult to evacuate. Early morning is often a good time to aim to have a regular bowel movement.

Other self-care activities in bowel management are an increased activity level—a sedentary lifestyle contributes to a slower passage of stool; a comfortable environment in which to move one's bowels rather than using a bedpan or a commode; and privacy in which to perform this hygienic function.

As mentioned earlier, certain medications for MS symptoms can adversely affect bowel function. These include antibiotics, anticholinergics, some antidepressants, and some binding agents used to control diarrhea. Antibiotics used to treat an infection can change the bacterial flora in the intestine, altering bowel patterns and increasing the production of intestinal flatus or gas.

Table 4.7   *Management of Bowel Problems*

General
- Maintain appropriate fluids (1.5–2 liters a day)
- Increase fiber in the diet (to 15 grams); daily intake should include:
  — One serving of fruit (with skin left on) or vegetable (served cooked, raw, or dried)
  — One-half to one serving of bread (whole wheat or rye) or fruit juice
  — One serving of bran (1 tablespoon), bran cereal, shredded wheat, nuts, or seeds; raw bran may be eaten plain, mixed with cereal, applesauce, soups, yogurt, or casseroles, or added to flour in cooking or baking.
- Try to have bowel movement at the same time every day
- Clean out all stool before starting a bowel regimen

Constipation
- Use 100% bran, prune juice, or other dietary triggers
- Over-the-counter laxatives
  — Bulk-forming agents
  — Fecal softeners
  — Stimulant cathartics
  — Suppositories (rectal stimulants)
  — Enemas
  — Saline cathartics
- Prescription medications

Diarrhea
- Monitor diet, weight, electrolyte loss
- Bulk-forming supplements
- Antidiarrheals
- Practice good skin care to avoid breakdown

Diarrhea is much less common than constipation. Dietary triggers should be sought, infection should be ruled out, and antidiarrheals may be used.

Uncontrolled bowel movements are treated by standardizing the bowel regimen to promote regular movements.

Dietary modifications can promote improved bowel function. Adequate fiber and bulk-producing food, adequate intake of fluids, and a regular meal pattern all contribute to effective bowel management (Table 4.7).

Sexual Problems

Normal sexual functioning involves a complex series of neurologically controlled events. As a result, up to 75 percent of men and 56 percent of women with MS may suffer from impaired sexual function. The physiologic responses to sexual arousal are mediated by the nervous system, so it is quite understandable that the disease can result in sexual dysfunction, either as an occasional problem or as an ongoing problem, depending on the specific clinical features of the disease. Men experience impotence and diminished libido. Women may suffer from vaginal dryness, diminished libido, *vaginismus* (painful tightening sensation in the vagina), and leg spasticity, which may lead to difficulty spreading the thighs. Incontinence of urine also is upsetting and inhibits most people from having spontaneous sexual activity. *Ataxia* (difficulty with balance) and weakness may make intercourse less satisfying, with orgasm difficult to achieve.

As with bowel and bladder dysfunction, the importance of sexual dysfunction should not be minimized. An approach to managing sexual dysfunction is outlined in Table 4.8. If one is experiencing this problem, the first step to treating it is to bring up the issue with the health care provider who is most involved in managing the MS. Management of erectile dysfunction has become easier during the past few years with the advent of sildenafil (Viagra®). For women, the ability to have sexual intercourse may be enhanced by using vaginal lubricants (Replens®, Astroglide®, KY® jelly), managing spasticity, and reducing bowel and bladder problems.

Beyond the physical issues of MS, there may be difficulty in achieving orgasm because of neurologic damage caused by MS. This is a difficult problem because it may also have an emotional component. Certainly, part of the treatment of sexual dysfunction should consist of counseling with someone who understands the issues. A problem-oriented treatment plan

Table 4.8 *Management of Sexual Problems*

- Discussions must include patient and partner
- Treat related problems (depression, pain, spasticity, fatigue)
- Alternate techniques
  — Displays of affection
  — Cuddling
  — Masturbation
  — Use of devices (vibrators, sex toys)
  — Changes in positioning
- Lubrication
- Erectile dysfunction
  — Sildenafil (Viagra®)
  — Penile injection
  — Urethral suppository (Muse®)
  — Inflatable and noninflatable penile implants
  — Vacuum suction (pump) devices

should be recommended for the psychological aspects of MS that affect sexuality and intimacy. This issue is discussed further in Chapter 8.

Skin Care

Inadequate skin care can lead to symptomatic problems in MS. An intact skin has four major functions: protection, sensory communication, temperature and fluid regulation, and fat and water storage. Taking care of your skin is as important as bladder and bowel management and overcoming other symptoms such as pain and fatigue. Skin breakdown can be a problem with worsening MS as the result of decreased mobility, diminished strength, and altered sensations. Your skin should be regularly inspected for breakdown. If redness occurs, *do not* massage the area because that will increase the risk of damage to underlying tissue. If the area remains red after you have changed position and removed the pressure, it is important to contact your health care professional. Similarly, if there is an opening in the skin, it should be promptly examined by a health care professional for prompt treatment.

The skin should be cleaned immediately when it is soiled. Waste products (stool and urine) can irritate the skin and cause skin breakdown. The use of warm water and a mild cleansing agent with a soft cloth will promote healthy tissue. Lubrication is also important; dry skin has greater potential for skin breakdown.

Key Points in Skin Care

- Keep your skin clean and dry.
- Do not remain in the same position for more than one hour.
- Report persistent irritations promptly.
- Learn ways to prevent and treat pressure sores.
- For those who are self-injecting: rotate sites regularly; examine injection sites before injecting; do not inject any area that is tender, hard, or discolored; and do not allow the medication to come in contact with the skin.

Pressure sores can be prevented by regular movement, shifting weight, changing position, doing chair pushups if upper extremity strength is adequate, practicing good skin care, relieving areas of pressure (using cushions or supports while sitting), using a special mattress to evenly distribute weight, protecting skin from injury, preventing incontinence, and developing good eating habits. If a pressure sore develops, prompt treatment is essential to prevent long-term complications of ongoing skin breakdown.

Depression

Until recently, depression in people with MS was thought to be a reaction to worsening of the disease. Based on more recent research, it is now believed that there may be a higher rate of mood disorders with this disease and that this increase may be the result of CNS damage and neurochemical changes caused by the disease. For example, psychiatric disturbances have been associated with lesions of the temporal lobe. Although the cause of depression remains unclear, certain genetic factors may be involved. It is possible that there are related genes that put one at risk for MS and depression. If depression does occur, one should talk about it with a physician, nurse, or counselor. It is important that effective treatment begin as soon as the problem is identified. Treatment may consist of counseling, medications, or a combination. If depression appears to be based on one's life situation, it may be necessary to focus on altering barriers and impediments to a desired quality of life.

The most important factor in managing depression is to acknowledge the problem and obtain treatment as quickly as possible. Health care providers should always be informed about the possibility of a mood disorder, in which case they may be interested in activities of daily living. The questions asked in the evaluation of depression may include the following:

- *Sleep:* Is there a change in sleep pattern? Insomnia or hypersomnia? Lack of ability to sleep or oversleepiness?
- *Interest:* Have you noticed that you are less interested in things that usually give you pleasure?
- *Guilt:* Do you think you are more guilty or remorseful than usual about things you have done or not done recently?
- *Energy:* Has there been a change in your energy level lately? (This is often difficult to assess in people with MS. It really should not be pivotal in deciding whether you are depressed.)
- *Concentration:* Do you find that your memory or concentration is less sharp than usual?
- *Appetite:* Has your appetite changed recently? Are you eating too much or too little?
- *Psychomotor:* Are you very agitated or very slow? Has your activity level changed from a normal pattern?
- *Suicide:* Have you thought that life is not worth living? Have you contemplated ending your life?

If four or more of these symptoms are present, it indicates to your physician or nurse that you may be depressed and require immediate intervention to elevate your mood. Unfortunately, there are few specific written guidelines for treating depression in MS. Studies indicate that treatment with psychotherapy or antidepressants usually reduces these symptoms. In general, optimal treatment for depression combines counseling and the use of an antidepressant (Table 4.9). Acknowledging depression and beginning treatment will undoubtedly promote lightened mood and a richer quality of life.

Other strategies that may help are participation in support groups, networking with others, and obtaining education and information about MS and its ramifications. A supportive social network is very beneficial to those living with the daily concerns about the disease and its ongoing problems.

Cognitive Dysfunction

A range of memory and other cognitive difficulties has been observed in people with MS. Functions that appear to be particularly affected are attention, memory (both short-term and long-term), information processing speed, abstract reasoning such as problem solving and conceptual reasoning, visuospatial perception, and learning ability. Many studies have demonstrated that 45 to 65 percent of people with MS have some degree of cognitive impairment but that only 10 percent are so impaired that it interferes with activities of daily living and work. Secondary progressive MS seems to be the subtype that is most associated with cognitive disturbances, and with longer duration of disease cognitive difficulties seem to occur more commonly in this group. In addition, cognitive deficits may occur and resolve in the same way other impairments do.

Cognitive dysfunction has little or no correlation with length or extent of disease, the extent of physical disability, or symptoms such as fatigue or depression. Significant relationships have been reported between cognitive deficits and changes in the brain on MRI imaging, particularly total lesion burden. Some investigators have found that there may be a link between the extent of MS lesions in the area of the brain called the *cerebrum* and poor

Table 4.9 *Management of Depression*

- Educate patient and family about warning signs
- Discuss the problem
- Consider psychotherapy
- Consider antidepressant therapy
- Monitor response to treatment at regular intervals

Table 4.10   *Management of Cognitive Problems*

- Identify the extent of the problem
  — Neurocognitive testing
- Discuss the problem: bring it out into the open
- Cognitive rehabilitation for coping/compensation strategies
- Consider medications

performance on cognitive testing. Cognitive evaluation or neuropsychological testing can provide the basis for management and counseling for those with this difficult symptom, with full feedback following the testing.

It is important to acknowledge and recognize cognitive dysfunction and move forward from there. Once the problem is identified, it is often a source of relief to those who have misinterpreted its effects as mental instability or a lack of caring about themselves. Each person's experience with cognitive dysfunction is unique and evolving. It is important to acknowledge the problem and develop some compensatory strategies: writing things down, keeping notes using a small handheld computer, and trying to establish routines may help to overcome problems with memory and judgment (Table 4.10).

Discussions with occupational therapists and physical therapists frequently help to develop strategies for safety, and repetition, along with written cues, will help embed them into memory. The availability of computers has certainly enhanced everyone's ability to function; people with MS may find a computer to be of great assistance in compensating for memory deficits. Medicines used for Alzheimer's disease have been tested in MS. In addition, the disease-modifying therapies may decrease the severity of cognitive difficulties. The emotional impact of cognitive impairment in MS cannot be underestimated, and a person who is experiencing these problems should be supported by the health care community, family members, and others who are providing counseling and educational services.

Summary

Symptomatic management and disease-modifying strategies provide the benchmarks of MS care. Appropriate management includes a wide variety of pharmacologic, nonpharmacologic, rehabilitative, and psychological approaches, as well as numerous self-care strategies. The issue in a progressive disease course is the restoration and maintenance of control of life-disrupting symptoms. By learning what to do and how to do it, you and your family can put MS in its "rightful place" and sustain an acceptable quality of life.

5

Facing the Challenge of Worsening Multiple Sclerosis: Tools for the Transition

The period when a person with multiple sclerosis (MS) realizes that he or she is getting worse is an extremely difficulty time. Facing disease progression is a *transition*, a change from the security of a full recovery from each attack to the accumulation of disabling symptoms and the increasing inability to be fully independent. The word *interdependence*—the need for support—enters one's vocabulary at that time. The use of assistive devices such as walkers, scooters, wheelchairs, equipment for activities of daily living, and environmental adaptations becomes a harsh reality of daily life. This period is truly a transition.

In reality, the initial diagnosis of MS is itself a transition, particularly in people who are young and relatively healthy. Once diagnosed, people with MS are suddenly thrust into a world of uncertainty in which they can no longer trust their bodies or the assurance of good health. They must also face the fact that MS is an unpredictable disease with variable effects. They become enmeshed in the health care system at a time when most people have little or no contact with physicians, nurses, or rehabilitation services. The other issue, of course, is the spectrum of changes that can result from this variable, perplexing, and dynamic disease. These changes can be physical, emotional, functional, intellectual, economic, and interpersonal. In facing worsening disease, people with MS must be empowered with *tools* for the transition—programs, services, information, and support that will help them adapt to change and remain functional and productive members of their families and the community in which they live. These tools can be classified as rehabilitative, psychosocial, and emotionally sustaining. The goal is to assist people with MS reestablish a harmony between their bodies and their "selves," a harmony that has been disrupted by the diagnosis of MS.

When people have mild disease or are in remission, the natural tendency is to want everything to remain the same or stay "normal"—the way things were before MS came along. In many respects, this is a very healthy response. But it involves a certain amount of denial, resistance to treatment, and effective life planning. People who feel fine do not want to think about the potential impact of MS on their future. The instinct of many is to put off dealing with issues such as rehabilitation and other types of services. As one begins to face a change in function, the integration and acceptance of change become a necessity in order to integrate new and necessary relationships and supports into daily living. Within recent years, the role of rehabilitation has taken a more predominant role in the spectrum of MS care.

Rehabilitation in Multiple Sclerosis

At one time or another during the course of the disease, rehabilitation may consist of contact with physiatrists, physical and occupational therapists, speech and language pathologists, and vocational and recreational specialists. The goal of rehabilitative services across the board is to promote maximal and safe functioning employing strategies, assistive devices, and effective energy expenditure. It is of primary important to define the roles of the various specialists that one sees in the rehabilitation setting.

Physiatrists are physicians who have specialized training in rehabilitation medicine. They are knowledgeable about physical and occupational therapy, as well as in the use of assistive devices to aid physically challenged patients. The specialty known as physiatry was founded by Dr. Howard Rusk in New York City during World War II, when many servicemen experienced disabling injuries during the war requiring services to allow them to return to fuller and more productive lives. Physiatrists care for patients in both inpatient and rehabilitation settings and in MS clinics and centers throughout the United States. They perform a comprehensive assessment to ascertain neurologic status, physical function, psychological adjustment, community supports, and the need for rehabilitative services. They work in close collaboration with the rehabilitation team to set achievable goals, assess outcomes, and plan for ongoing programs, services, and modifications, both personal and environmental.

Physical therapists (PTs) treat problems involving ambulation, balance, coordination, strength, and mobility. They provide services and education to strengthen muscles, teach the appropriate use of rehabilitation equipment and mobility devices, measure for and apply braces and other orthotic supports, and guide people to maintain a fitness-oriented lifestyle. Physical therapists emphasize the delicate balance between exercise and fatigue and can be helpful in suggesting the most appropriate recreational activities. The assessment by a PT includes muscle strength, range of motion, proprioception (the perception of your location in space—is the toe up or down, etc.), muscle tone, gait, balance, transfers, and mobility.

Occupational therapists (OTs) deal with energy conservation issues, activities of daily living, upper extremity function, sitting balance, wheelchair selection and cushions, and other mobility devices. They are knowledgeable about aids to daily living and modifications in the home environment: bathrooms, kitchens, entrances and stairways, and motor vehicles. Occupational therapists also assist people to remain at work by recommending changes in the work environment. The focus of an OT is to improve the quality of a person's life by developing or maintaining those abilities that are essential to productive living. An OT evaluation should be done initially and repeated every 6 to 12 months to assess for change. The assessment should include current living situation and responsibilities, vocational status, hand dominance (which hand the patient thinks is more functional and whether this has changed since the onset of the disease), previous therapy, adaptive equipment used, and ambulation status. Additionally, there are formal tests of grip and pinch, coordination, and activities of daily living.

Speech and language pathologists (SLPs) work with people who are having problems with breathing, swallowing, speech, and cognition. These therapists teach people to overcome these deficits through exercises and other compensatory strategies. Modern technology may be incorporated into therapy sessions (computers, communication devices). A clinical speech/swallowing and mental status assessment can be accomplished in approximately one hour. Best results are achieved when the person being tested is well rested. The assessment will include speech, an oral peripheral examination, and the adequacy of facial or mouth structures. In addition, speech quality will be assessed: sustained speech, counting on one breath, reading, and spontaneous conversation. The swallowing assessment will focus on the severity of the swallowing problem, types of food or fluid that cause the problem, and taste. Foods such as nectar, peaches, crackers, puddings, and water may be used for a swallowing evaluation. If complex problems are identified, a swallow study using an X-ray may be prescribed. This study, (a modified *barium swallow*) will allow the therapist to determine which consistency of food causes the most difficulty and will then result in an individualized plan of care for food preparation and eating. Speech and language pathologists also evaluate people for language, cognitive, or memory deficits.

Recreational therapists (RTs) help people with MS to find diverse activities that are appropriate to their level of functioning and give them a quality of life beyond the work-a-day world. They allow an expansion of daily activities to provide creative and enjoyable outlets. Activities such as swimming, yoga, tai chi, hippotherapy (horseback riding), meditation, and other fitness programs have been found beneficial in MS. Reading, computer use, board games, and other mind-stimulating programs are very important for recreation with others and for relaxation.

The delivery of rehabilitation services can be done in many venues: at home, in outpatient facilities, in inpatient programs, in health clubs and gyms, and within MS centers. The approach to MS rehabilitation must be quite different from how an orthopedic patient with a fracture or a spinal cord injured person receives care. The issue of fatigue affects the pace of rehabilitation. Many people with other diseases can take two to four hours of rehabilitation. People with MS may have problems dealing with that type of schedule. It is very important to establish an appropriate exercise and condition program that will not allow fatigue to interfere with function. Teaching energy conservation and pacing early becomes very valuable.

When is rehabilitation indicated in MS? Certainly, it is appropriate during an acute exacerbation that has produced a significant change in functions such as walking, coordination, strength, or stamina. Rehabilitation in the context of an acute attack usually is time-limited and goal-oriented—the aim is to return to a prior level of function. Rehabilitation also is indicated during disease progression, when one is gradually losing function and is no longer able to move and transfer safely or be as mobile as in the past. A program at that time may consist of professional services along with self-care activities such as a home exercise program, aquatherapy, or a personal fitness program at a gymnasium or health club. Studies have indicated that a targeted rehabilitation program can improve not only strength of weakened muscles but also MS-related fatigue, depression, and social isolation.

It is important to remember that the duration of rehabilitation services will depend not only on available personnel and facilities but also on third-party reimbursement (insurance coverage). Most insurance carriers require that rehabilitation prescriptions contain information about desired outcomes—goals of therapy and specific benchmarks (i.e., ambulation with a walker, ability to walk 50 feet, safe transfers, etc.). Once these goals have been achieved, rehabilitation usually is terminated, with potential for reassessment once additional rehabilitation goals can be identified.

Tools for the Transition

People with progressive MS generally have ongoing walking, coordination, and balance problems. They are subject to falls and other accidents within the home or in the workplace. It is important to use appropriate assistive equipment. These are tools not only to assist in energy conservation but also to promote safe and effective mobility, including transfers, and improve independence.

Tools for the transition to progressive MS include many assistive devices: adapted utensils with large cushion grips to make them easier to handle; scooters (three-wheeled motorized carts), lightweight wheelchairs, wheeled walkers, shower chairs, tub seats, bathtub handrails, safety mats, and personal hygiene equipment, to name only a few (Table 5.1).

In addition, plate guards help keep food on the plate when there is only the use of one hand or a minimal use of the other hand. A mug that is easy to hold may not require a fine grip but will allow someone to drink a full cup of coffee. A buttonhook can allow someone to put on a dress shirt in the morning and button it in 5 minutes instead of 30 minutes. There are many types of writing devices that make handwriting more intelligible and reduce fatigue. A kitchen stool will allow a homemaker to prepare and cook meals without prolonged standing. The same stool will allow the person with MS to assist with washing dishes, folding laundry, and ironing, thus participating in the chores at home.

For those with speech difficulties, communication can be facilitated by adapted computers. Voice recognition can support someone with a severe tremor who is unable to manipulate a mouse or a keyboard. Multiple adaptive keypads are available for the visually impaired.

Speech therapists can teach people with swallowing problems new strategies for safe eating. A number of products are available or can be adapted to promote a nutritious diet. Puréed foods and products that thicken liquids are readily available for this problem.

Recreational activities can be adapted to changing physical capabilities. There is no reason a person with MS should not have a full social life. Thanks to the Americans with Disabilities Act, most public facilities

Table 5.1   *Tools for Ambulation*

Assistive Device	Parameters for Use	Rehabilitation Interventions
Crutches Forearm	Full use of upper extremities Weakness in legs	Proper use of crutches Gait training/transfer training Safety measures
Canes Quad Tripod Straight	Good arm strength Balance problems Weakness in one leg	Gait training Transfer training Safety measures
Walker	Generalized weakness in both legs Good arm strength	Gait training Transfer training Safety measures
Wheelchair	Diminished stamina Fatigue Weakness in legs and/or arms or inability to walk	Proper measurement of chair Assessment where used Modifications for home and/or work Specific weight for person's strength Wheelchair cushion *Possible modifications* High back Reclining back Removable arms or leg rests Elevating swingaway leg rests Head and neck support Can be manual or motorized Can be propelled electrically with a joystick or mouthpiece Should be transportable in a van or car
Motorized tricart or scooter	Fatigue Need to walk long distances Unable to propel manual wheelchair	Proper measurement Assessment where used Appropriate size and modifications for person's dimensions

have been adapted to suit the needs of people with disabilities. Restaurants, theaters, parks, and sports arenas have modified entrances and lavatory facilities to accommodate people who use a wheelchair or other mobility device.

Psychosocial Issues in Disease Progression

What happens in a person with progressive MS? There are more frequent telephone calls to the health care provider with ongoing problems. The person with MS encounters increasing difficulties in taking care of himself or herself and begins to have problems managing day-to-day activities. This may be due to a physical accumulation of problems as well as cognitive changes. Symptoms become more persistent.

People at this point in the transition require a great deal of reassurance and support. This poses a great burden on family members and close significant others. People who are in a transitional period of their disease have a keen sense of what is going on. They realize that there is change, and they may be frightened. These changes may present subtly at first, but with time there may be more impairment and disability. The challenge is to work with the changes to adapt to the dynamic, continually changing situation provoked by progressive disease.

There is no cookbook recipe for dealing with worsening MS—there is no one drug or management strategy. The challenge for this period is to sustain therapies, medications, and self-care activities that will control and reduce symptoms, prevent injury, and sustain necessary supports. Programs and services must be adapted to individual and family needs with consideration of ethnic, social, and economic background. During the past decade, it has become obvious that deconditioning as a result of sustained rest and inactivity is detrimental. It is important to maintain cardiovascular and respiratory fitness for physical wellness. In the psychological realm, it is equally important for a person to remain productive and involved in daily activities. This can be difficult in our society, in which productivity is equated with physical action. People with progressive MS must redefine productivity in the context of their changing lives. Although a person with MS may not be able to go out and play baseball with her children or be a soccer mom, productivity may just involve being there when her children are doing their homework or playing games. A person with worsening MS needs to seek alternative methods for feeling worthwhile, communicating needs, and feeling like part of his or her family.

Adaptability and flexibility are important personal characteristics as one learns to deal with change. Those of us who are parents can remember the times we have said "I will never have a teen phone in my house" or "I will never give my son or daughter the car." As children age, that boundary suddenly has to shift—when the 13-year-old monopolizes the telephone for hours or when the teenager has after-school activities and Mom or Dad are very tired. It is important to acknowledge that flexibility does not signify weakness of character or "giving in" to the children.

Adapting to worsening disease should also include a sense of realistic hope about the future—as Dr. Rosalind Kalb has said, "planning for the worst, while hoping for the best." Realistic hope is contingent upon education about MS, available therapies, and reasonable expectations about outcomes. Realistic expectations have a positive impact not only on hope, but also on adherence to any therapy throughout a lifetime with this disease.

The important message for anyone with progressive MS is to normalize your lifestyle whenever possible, to minimize energy expenditure, and to establish a desirable as well as a safe quality of life. While rehabilitation in MS cannot be restorative, it has the primary aim of maintenance of function, prevention of deterioration, and safety. This hopeful philosophy—this wellness model—has an important message for those with progressive disease: to use all the tools and supports available at this time and throughout the rest of your life with MS.

6

Increasing Disability: Social and Economic Issues

Based on the variability of the disease course and the intermittent nature of symptoms, it is not surprising that multiple sclerosis (MS) has a pervasive social and economic impact. From the time of diagnosis throughout the course of the disease, it is important to assess and reassess current status, adapt to changing circumstances, and maintain a productive and full quality of life. This process can be facilitated by anticipatory planning with your "MS team"—family, friends, colleagues, and health care providers. You can also obtain support from community organizations such as the National MS Society, clergy, personnel who specialize in vocational rehabilitation, and other organizations that represent individuals who are disabled or chronically ill.

As MS progresses, symptoms may become ongoing, more intense, and more disabling. The performance of activities of daily living, social activities, and paid work may suffer. Personal development and long-term plans may undergo radical changes. From the perspective of careers, the most active decades of growth are those in which MS is usually diagnosed (20–40 years). During this period, people become established in their careers and continue in activities that lead to the attainment of lifetime goals. People with progressive MS may find themselves facing a slowing of career development. In many cases, there may be a loss of career altogether. Ninety percent of Americans with MS have been employed, and approximately 60 percent are employed at the time of diagnosis. However, the

National Multiple Sclerosis Society reports that only 25 percent of people with MS in the United States are employed in the years after diagnosis. Why does this occur? Several factors have been linked to MS patients' employment status, including gender, socioeconomic status, and age.

Gender

Gender is a major unemployment factor for people with MS. Women are significantly less likely to be employed than men. This seems to be a consistent pattern in both the United States and Canada. A recent national survey in the United States revealed unemployment rates of 84 percent for women compared with 72 percent for men. Canada shows a similar disparity in employment based on gender. Although mobility impairment is a strong predictor of job loss for men, severe physical symptoms such as bladder and bowel dysfunction and debilitating fatigue predict job loss for women. In a 1986 study, a lower level of education was associated with unemployment among men with MS but not among women.

Socioeconomic Status

Both men and women with MS are more likely to leave the work force if they have a spouse who is working, they have high levels of education, and/or they have substantial money in savings and investments. This finding might be explained by suggesting that people with higher levels of education tend to have better financial resources.

Many people with MS who have the financial means to stop working do so voluntarily and are unlikely to return. Many factors may contribute to this decision, one of which might be health insurance coverage. Under the previous law, disabled people often lost Medicaid and Medicare coverage because their income increased when they returned to work. In December 1999 President Clinton signed the Work Incentives Improvement Act, which expands Medicaid and Medicare so that people with disabilities can continue to receive health insurance coverage once they return to work. This law, with provisions that will be phased in, provides $150 million for grants to encourage states to allow disabled workers to buy into Medicaid, paying premiums in amounts that would be largely left up to the states. It also sets aside funds to help obtain Medicaid coverage for people who are minimally disabled but cannot work—those with a progressive disease. Perhaps these trends will be reversed in the future based on this much needed change in the law.

Age

Middle-aged people with MS more often remain employed compared with the younger and older MS population. Two factors help to explain why this happens. First, there is a significant relationship between age and MS-related physical disability. Older people with MS typically have a longer disease duration and are more likely to have a progressive course. Accumulated disability tends to increase with disease progression, thus restricting the ability of a worker to meet the physical demands of his or her job. Second, older people tend to have the financial means to stop working and do so to focus on other aspects of their lives. On the other hand, younger people may not have had the opportunity for skills development or accrual of adequate experience to obtain and sustain paid employment. Therefore, the younger segment of the MS population may be found on the disability rolls because they have not had the opportunity to establish themselves in the work force.

What Can Be Done to Help?

People with progressive MS face a life of ongoing challenges and uncertainty. They also are presented with a variety of options to sustain their productivity within the work force. The Americans with Disabilities Act (ADA) of 1990 was the most significant piece of legislation for this segment of the population in decades. Implicit in the ADA was the guarantee of equal rights in society for all people with disabilities, both in day-to-day living and in employment. The implementation of the ADA is the responsibility of employers, government officials, and people with MS. The ADA has implications for the workplace, social gatherings, the community, and educational settings. It can affect a person's ability to remain a productive member of the work force. Those people facing a transition in their MS should avail themselves of the benefits of this legislation.

Job Modifications

In general, job retention activities for people with disabilities are most effective when a priority is placed on helping the person continue in his or her current position through a variety of programs and services. The term *reasonable accommodation* is used in this context. Reasonable accommodation may consist of installing new equipment such as voice-activated computers, restructuring job responsibilities, modifying work schedules, revamping workspace for wheelchair accessibility, changing the location of the worksite to include telecommuting (working at home with a computer), reassignment to another position, providing personal and professional assistance, or modifying the workspace to accommodate assistive devices such as walkers or wheelchairs.

The first step to initiate reasonable accommodation is to approach your supervisor or human resources person to discuss your needs and concerns. This step engages both the employee and the employer in the process of examining the issues related to job performance and job retention. Discussions should include information related to your position and the requirements related to job responsibilities. It may involve physical and cognitive aspects of your job as well as the support systems needed to maximize your role. It is also important to openly discuss barriers to successful job performance.

Future plans should include assistance that will meet both your needs and those of your employer in terms of job modifications, adjustments, or accommodations that will promote the achievement and maintenance of satisfactory work performance. State vocational rehabilitation services may be engaged in this process by providing both technical services and direct support. Vocational rehabilitation services include education to facilitate career changes, facilitation of telecommuting programs, vehicle modification with hand controls, and career counseling for those people unsure of future direction. The goal of vocational rehabilitation service programs is to facilitate job retention, return to the work force, or retraining for more appropriate careers. People with MS should use these services and take advantage of the expertise and experience that may help them.

Getting Around

Diminished mobility may be a major consequences of MS and may involve walking, transferring, bed mobility, and driving. As discussed earlier in the chapter on rehabilitation, people with disease progression require intermittent and individualized attention to their changing mobility needs. The key is to maintain safety and facilitate maximal independence. Just as assistive devices may be used as tools for the transition, vehicular modifications will promote maximal transportation to and from work and other desired activities. Hand controls in an automobile allow the driver to maneuver a vehicle safely and efficiently without excessive fatigue. Controls are placed on the steering wheel and alongside the steering post to allow for turning, acceleration, deceleration, and braking. Many people participate in a pre-driving evaluation by a trained professional who checks hand–eye coordination, depth perception, reflexes, and reaction time to determine whether it is safe to drive and what modifications are advisable. Trunk lifts, roof racks, and special swivel seats may facilitate safe driving.

If a person with MS is working, the office of vocational rehabilitation may financially support vehicular modifications if he or she is eligible for these services. For people who are nonambulatory, modified vans with lifts and wheelchair tie-down equipment are another option for transportation.

Getting around in cities and in the suburbs may be challenging for someone with a disability. Title II of the ADA covers public transportation, including city bus, rail, ferries, subways, Amtrak, and commuter rail. The key point is that public transportation cannot discriminate against people with disabilities, and transportation services for those unable to use regular carrier systems must be made available. Paratransit may include small van and taxi services. In rail services at least one car per train must be accessible to people who use a wheelchair.

Using Public Accommodations

The 1990 ADA requires that people with medical problems such as MS have access to public accommodations, including buildings operated by state and local government agencies or private owners who open buildings to the public. Access requirements are intended to ensure the full participation of people with disabilities. Older buildings must be modified or programs moved to make them accessible to the public; new buildings must comply with standards for accessibility. The ADA prohibits discrimination on the basis of disability in public accommodations and commercial facilities. This includes businesses, restaurants, medical offices, theaters, private schools, museums, sports arenas, day care centers, and retail stores, to name but a few. Hotels, motels, and inns are general covered with an exception for small lodgings such as bed-and-breakfasts. Every public or common-use bathroom must have at least one stall that is accessible; two, if there are six or more stalls. The basic goal of these provisions is that architectural barriers must be removed in existing facilities unless doing so would be an undue burden. New or altered facilities must comply with the ADA Accessibility Guidelines.

Your Legal Rights

Getting around today also means having access to communication devices and other technology designed to help those with chronic illnesses or disabilities. The ADA deals with telephone and television access for people with vision or hearing impairments and stipulates that phone companies must establish 24-hour-a-day 7-day-a-week interstate and intrastate communications relay services. This is to allow communication with people who use regular voice phones.

The right to access for people with disabilities is not limited to access to technological services or building design, particularly in governmental or tax-supported agencies. Programs and activities for the general population must demonstrate reasonable accommodation for those with disabilities and must be provided in an integrated setting. Safety requirements may be imposed if they are necessary for the safe provision of services, but they must be based on objective standards. Emergency services must provide access for people with a disability, but there is no requirement that wheelchairs, glasses, attendants, or other personal assistance be required.

A state or local government may choose to provide additional services or benefits, but people with MS can opt not to use them. Churches, clubs, and private organizations are not covered under the ADA, although they may be subject to state statutes if they are available for use by the general public.

Housing

The Fair Housing Amendments Act (FHAA) of 1988 prohibits discrimination in housing based on family status and handicap. This was an expansion of the protections of the Fair Housing Act of 1968, which banned discrimination on the basis of race, color, national origin, religion, or sex, and on Section 504 of the Rehabilitation Act of 1973, which prohibited discrimination on the basis of disability. Under the FHAA, no one can refuse to sell, rent, or make available a house, apartment, or other dwelling on the basis of a buyer's or renter's handicap. It also is illegal to discriminate on the basis of the handicap of someone associated with a buyer or renter, as when a spouse is physically disabled with MS.

Much of the housing in the United States is covered by the FHAA, but single-family homes that are privately sold are exempted from its provisions. Nothing in the FHAA requires the seller of the single-family home to make the house accessible. However, in the case of a rental, a landlord cannot prevent a person with a disability from making reasonable modifications for his or her own use and at his or her own expense. Such modifications must be done so that the property can be restored to its original condition at the expiration of the lease. A landlord may ask a tenant to provide a description of the work to be done, along with reasonable assurance that it will be carried out in a legal fashion. A landlord may not increase the rent or demand increased security as a condition for modifications but may require an agreement in writing to ensure restoration of the property. This may include an amount of money sufficient to cover restoration costs with accrued interest given to the tenant.

Filing for Disability

Anyone who has been diagnosed with MS should be aware of disability benefits available from the Social Security Administration (SSA), private disability insurance, or coverage from an employer. The first decision to be made when considering work status is to be certain that it is appropriate to stop working. Each person must evaluate his or her own condition in consultation with the family, physician, or significant people at work. In addition, it might be wise to investigate alternatives to long-term retirement—part-time work, telecommuting, and so forth. It is also appropriate to work with vocational counselors, teachers, and employment agencies to determine whether current work remains an option or if other alternatives may be viable in light of the functional impairments imposed by MS.

Once a person files for disability, it is not an easy task to return to work. This is a pivotal decision in one's life and must not be taken lightly. To receive long-term disability compensation, a number of steps must be followed and a great deal of paperwork is involved. Length of time worked, salary, and time span between onset of illness or disability are factors involving in obtaining coverage. For further information on this topic, readers are referred to *Multiple Sclerosis: Your Legal Rights*, by Lanny and Sara Perkins (see "Additional Readings"). This book is an excellent resource for information on long-term disability and health insurance issues.

Health Insurance

The first step in self-education about insurance is to determine your coverage and eligibility status. If you are employed, what are your benefits? What is covered and what is not? Read your employee manuals, written brochures, and other information related to your coverage. It is important to have an actual copy of your policy so that you can understand your coverage. It is also important to understand whether you have a prescription plan and whether a copayment (money you must pay when you visit a doctor or obtain your medications) is required.

If you are not employed and you want to obtain insurance, how can you manage this with a diagnosis of MS? Many states have laws that require health insurance providers to have periods of open enrollment during which anyone with a preexisting condition may buy a policy. This may be the best way to get affordable coverage. Professional, academic, and social organizations also may offer affordable plans. Benefits and other features such as a waiting period or exclusions for preexisting conditions must be analyzed. Is there a cap on how much coverage is provided? Does it offer all the benefits you may need?

One method of researching insurance questions is to contact your state board of insurance, insurance commission, or similar government office. Again, *Multiple Sclerosis: Your Legal Rights* is an excellent resource for a comprehensive overview of health insurance, as is *Insurance Solutions: Plan Well, Live Better* by Laura Cooper (see "Additional Readings").

Managed Care

In many states, more than 85 percent of people who receive coverage from their employers are enrolled in a managed care plan. There are two types of managed care organizations: HMOs (health maintenance organizations) and PPOs (preferred provider organizations). With an HMO, out-of-pocket fees are minimal but the choice of health care provider is limited. In a PPO, there is a larger panel of providers and more liberal access to care.

Managed care has frequently posed problems for people with MS by placing limitations on specialist visits or care at MS specialty centers. If you are enrolled in a managed care program, there may come a time when you have to consider paying additional medical costs out of pocket to continue with your specialty program or to secure treatments that may not be covered through the managed care system. The National MS Society's Clinical Program Department can assist people with MS to navigate the complex contemporary health care system and advocate for needed programs and services.

Federal Programs

Those with progressive disease and substantial disability who apply for and receive Social Security benefits will be eligible to receive Medicare benefits after two years. It might be advisable to investigate Medicare managed care options and/or supplemental insurance. Fortunately, Medicare supplements must now be standardized so that purchasers can more easily compare policies. However, not all plans are available in all states.

While Medicare offers coverage to those who qualify for disability benefits, Medicaid is offered only to those whose earnings qualify them for county and state medical assistance. People with MS who have served in the military should check with the Department of Veterans Affairs (VA) to see if they are eligible for disability, health, or life insurance; home modification; equipment; transportation; or other benefits. Many requirements influence the granting of VA benefits, including the period served, length of service, percentage of disability, sources of income, discharge status, and date of onset of illness. The general rule regarding MS coverage during "time of war" is that it must be demonstrated that at least a 10 percent disability was in evidence within 10 years of the date of discharge.

Coping with Taxes

Taxes affect every aspect of our lives, and those with MS are not exempt from this concern. While a person is working, earned income is taxed as usual. Once a person is either on temporary or long-term disability and is receiving a disability pension, this income will be taxable if the premiums for the disability insurance were paid by the employer. The pension may not be taxable if you obtained the policy as an individual and you paid the premiums (see *Insurance Solutions: Plan Well, Live Better* by Laura Cooper). In some instances, a person with MS may be eligible for a tax break on small amounts of the disability pension if there is no other income.

Once you qualify for Social Security disability payments, these payments will not be taxable unless you have income from another source such as a spouse's job or investments. An accountant will be able to advise your family about these matters, tax deductions related to MS-expenses, and other itemized deductions. There are many legal tax supports for people with disabilities that can be explained to you by a qualified accountant who is familiar with this type of tax law. For example, a certain portion of air-conditioning in one's home can be deductible as a medically necessary modification if you have a heat-sensitive condition such as MS. There are numerous other related medical expenses that can be enumerated for you and your family when you are confronted with disease progression and increased financial outlay as a result.

Personal Choices and Long-Term Planning

People with MS, as most people, want to make their own decisions about business affairs, lifestyle choices, and property for as long as possible. As the disease becomes progressive and the effects of physical changes increase (diminished mobility, altered stamina, and changes in the ability to perform activities of daily living), one needs to make provisions—both formal and informal—to ensure that important activities continue uninterrupted. For example, banks, mortgage companies, and other important institutions involved in daily living may need to be notified that future transactions will be handled by mail, telephone, or computer. These organizations often will be very cooperative if this plan is explained in advance. The Internet and catalogs may be helpful in dealing with important activities that may be curtailed by limited mobility.

If MS continues to progress and vision problems and other limitations interfere with the normal conduct of business or personal affairs, you may designate a trusted individual to act on your behalf through a *power of attorney*. This is a formal legal document that designates a family member, friend, or significant other to take actions such as signing documents, making decisions regarding expenditures, or the buying or selling of property. A power of attorney may be "general," which gives the person a very wide authority, or it can be a "special power of attorney," which authorizes him or her to take only a particular action or deal with a specific piece of business. Both types of powers of attorney may be revoked or assigned to another person. *It is advisable not to give irrevocable power of attorney to anyone unless you are well advised by a lawyer.*

The type of powers of attorney that people with MS are most interested in frequently are those that deal specifically with health care issues. These powers have names such as "durable power of attorney for health care," "health care proxy," "advanced directive for health care," or "medical directive." Their purpose is to appoint another person to make medical treatment decisions for you if you are unable to do so yourself. Numerous forms and documents are available through hospitals, other health care facilities, and organizations representing the chronically ill and disabled, but it is advisable to seek counsel from legal authorities because each state controls what is enforceable under these instruments.

Ultimately, all of us will face death. A "living will" or "directive to physicians" describes your wishes in the event that you are comatose or terminally ill. This is the manner in which one informs a physician or family about a person's wishes about food, water, or other medical care when death appears imminent. State laws also control this type of document.

For both kinds of directives, it is important not only to seek legal counsel but also to discuss your wishes with your family or close friends so that they are clear about treatment desires. Some states have *surrogate* laws that establish a hierarchy of people (spouses, parents, adult children, etc.) who may make treatment decisions for a person if he or she is unable to do so. Obviously, planning ahead, designating an agent, and having open discussions establish a clear plan for end-of-life decisions.

Trusts

Facing the progression of MS forces you to make long-term decisions regarding finances. You may choose to have a "trust" set up to sustain an ongoing income without having to deal with the details of investing or managing money. A trust agreement is drawn up by an attorney designating someone as the trustee, whose job it becomes to make those decisions. As the term implies, the trustee should be a *trusted* person, whether a family member or an outsider, but also someone who is knowledgeable about handling money. Although a trust is generally created for long periods of time, it can be *revocable* or *irrevocable* as determined by the person with the contract.

Along with a power of attorney, a trust may circumvent the need for a court-appointed guardianship or conservatorship, which usually are expensive and cumbersome. Certain trusts, sometimes called *supplemental needs trusts*, may protect assets while permitting eligibility for government programs such as Medicaid. Trusts, estates, and government benefits are highly technical areas of the law that require knowledgeable and experienced specialists. Therefore, it is important to work with experts in this field for this important activity related to progressive disease and its implications.

Conclusion

Multiple sclerosis results in many symptoms, many losses, and numerous changes in one's life. The uncertainty of when and how relapses may occur—and how fully one will recover—demands flexibility and an unusual level of coping. The prospect of disease progression presents the person and the family with additional challenges. These challenges can be met with a variety of strategies and supports that are available to those affected by the disease over a lifetime.

7

Coping with Disease Progression

*H*ow do people adjust to multiple sclerosis (MS)? Your emotional reactions and the reactions of your family members will ebb and flow with changes in the illness. Each attack and each new symptom or change in function will require that you readjust all over again. This may be a tiring process. The goal of emotional adjustment is not only to promote total acceptance but also to adapt to the presence of MS in daily living (see Kalb in "Additional Readings"). This requires making room for the disease without giving it more space, more time, or more energy than it absolutely needs.

From the time of diagnosis, the psychoeducational approach offers both education and counseling. It is designed to help the person with MS to cope, self-manage, problem-solve, and plan as comfortably and effectively as possible. It is important to be as alert to emotional and cognitive changes as you are to physical changes. Memory problems, word-finding difficulty, slowed processing speed, mood swings, and even depression can be among the initial symptoms and can occur in anyone with MS, regardless of the degree of physical impairment.

These changes need prompt attention not only because they are painful and difficult to live with, but also because they have an impact on how you spend your days. These symptoms will determine your ability to learn, develop problem-solving strategies, and initiate self-care activities. It also is important to remember that certain medications may affect emotions and cognition, so it would be appropriate to call a physician or a nurse about these concerns. For example, glucocorticoids (e.g., prednisone, methylprednisolone, dexamethasone), which are commonly used to manage clinical exacerbations, can wreck havoc on a person's emotions and contribute to emotional upheaval.

Some typical reactions to the diagnosis of MS include: "This can't be happening to me!" (denial); "What else is going to happen to me?" (anxiety); "Why can't you fix it?" (anger); and "At least I have a name for it!" (relief). From the time of the beginning of the disease throughout a lifetime with it, people will experience periods of grief and loss. Every new symptom, every new attack, and each new medication may represent a loss of certainty and control or loss of a particular skill or ability. Each adult spends a lifetime building a picture of himself or herself. As this picture changes, the person needs to grieve before reassembling the pieces and organizing a new self-image.

For the person with complete recovery after an exacerbation, a certain unreality sets in—the feeling that this was all a mistake, a bad dream, or something that can be conquered. The second attack, or the onset of progressive disease, brings home the reality of the illness, particularly in light of the recent emphasis on early intervention. Many people react by saying "I feel fine! Why should I give myself a shot?" or "What good will it do? I am getting worse anyway." It is important to view injectable therapy as a tool to regain and maintain control, an instrument to use on your own behalf, or a skill with which you can take charge of the unwelcome guest that is MS.

Unpredictability and loss of control can make people with MS and their families angry and resentful. Anger can be the greatest problem because people with MS have difficulty understanding what to do with it and how to express it. It is important to channel anger and to express it in a constructive way—not at each other, but at the disease itself. People with MS may feel anger in general; it is important that one not be afraid to express these feelings without the fear of driving away a care partner. Each one of us needs an outlet—talking, doing, and communicating, both verbally and nonverbally.

People with MS also experience a great deal of guilt, which may have to do with a real or perceived inability to fulfill roles and responsibilities in different areas of life. People worry that they are letting others down, that they are not "carrying their own weight." There may be guilt over these feelings as well. With disease progression, there may be a greater temptation to veer away from standard treatments and to try alternative means of managing the illness. At this time, there is a great need for education and support from health care providers, support groups, and local MS Society chapters.

The transition to disease progression represents a sometimes devastating loss of control; symptoms that were merely sporadic annoyances become lasting impediments that interfere with activities and threaten role performance in the home, at work, and in the community. Many people become "depressed" at this time. What is depression? Depression can be a brief reaction to a situation, or it can become clinical depression. What is it?

Clinical depression is different from normal grieving. It has a specific diagnostic criteria and requires medical intervention. Features that suggest clinical depression include:

■ Feeling depressed most of the day
■ Diminished interest or pleasure in everything
■ Significant weight change, up or down
■ Sleep disturbance, difficulty falling asleep or staying asleep, or early morning awakening
■ Motor slowing or motor agitation
■ Fatigue
■ Feelings of guilt or worthlessness
■ An inability to think or concentrate

Treatment usually consists of a medication called an antidepressant along with supportive counseling. The goal of treatment is to address the whole person and his and her living situation. Although most depressive episodes usually resolve with this therapy, the time to resolution varies from person to person (see Chapter 4).

As impairments begin to accumulate and disability creeps into more areas of daily life, people may attribute other meanings to the changes—"I must not be trying hard enough," "I am not praying enough," "I may not be exercising enough." One should understand that disease progression is not something that you can control voluntarily; there is little reason for guilt or self-blame. A person experiencing this problem needs support and the time and opportunity to express these feelings to people who can provide that support.

There is also the issue of cognitive changes related to MS. These changes may be relatively mild and amenable to remedial interventions and compensatory strategies (see Chapter 4). More severe deficits occur in a small percentage of people with the disease, and these can significantly interfere with the ability to function in life roles. In the past, people with MS, their family members, and even health care providers have been reluctant to talk about this problem. Fortunately, this is improving as our understanding of

MS is expanding. There is more information about the cognitive implications of MS and increasing research in this area.

Disease progression usually translates in a number of ways: progressive loss of abilities, activities, and life roles. But with progression can also come personal growth and the development of new skills. Although disease progression can be painful, it can be challenging as well. There is grief in dealing with both loss and change, but there also is the opportunity to reassess how one wishes to spend the rest of one's life. The psychosocial challenges that confront the person with progressive disease include finding new personal meaning for the concepts of self, independence, and control; finding the part of himself or herself that MS cannot touch; and identifying new goals and areas of focus.

For example, a person who becomes increasingly dependent on a variety of assistive devices and personal aids, outside assistance, and environmental modifications needs to take pride and satisfaction in being able to identify, obtain, and manage these resources. It is important to find new ways to think about exerting independence, being interdependent with others, and maintaining control of daily life, even though it may feel as if others are in control physically. Even those who are more disabled and who feel that every aspect of their lives has been affected by MS or that their life space has become constricted by disease-related limitations should seek a personal "MS-free zone," a place where the disease cannot reach. For one person it may be reading, music, or using a computer; for another, religious activities or community programs. It is important to look inside oneself to find an emotional respite from the disease and its day-to-day challenges. This respite reenergizes a person and "refuels" one's emotional reserves.

The person with progressive MS needs to redefine his or her self-image, make different plans, and identify new ways of feeling useful and productive. Counseling can be particularly helpful at this time to support your efforts to deal with painful feelings. Counseling can also assist by teaching you how to communicate effectively with others, think through a problem to find a solution, and keep up with the pace of the world in which you live.

Caregiver issues come to the fore with progressive disability. The families that seem to cope most effectively are those that develop a care partnership. While the person with MS may need new and different types of care as the disease progresses, the needs of the well spouse remain important as well. The couple in this partnership must find ways to meet each other's needs, to collaborate on planning and decision making, and to share the challenges. Progressive MS confronts a couple's emotional and physical intimacy in a variety of ways, the most obvious being the sexual changes that often occur with the disease (see Chapter 8).

In addition to the physical changes, emotional and attitudinal problems often accompany role shifts within families. Many well spouses may discuss how difficult it is to feel sexual attraction toward a person who functions in a very different role in their partnership than was previously the case or one who requires a great deal of intimate, hands-on care. Fatigue, experienced by both the person with MS and the care partner, may contribute to the feeling that sex is the last thing on anyone's mind. The most insidious challenge to a couple's intimacy comes from unexpressed feelings, mood changes, and cognitive problems.

People with severe disability are called upon to make important life decisions at a time when they are least equipped to do so. The quality of the partnership before and during the illness, the support programs that are provided to the couple, and the nature of the care that is available to those affected by progressive MS are important factors in strengthening and sustaining relationships and partnerships.

Conclusion

People with progressive MS may perceive their world to be shrinking and their options to be disappearing. Education, counseling, and support are needed on an ongoing basis; solutions to problems must be identified; priorities must be rearranged; and new and meaningful life options must be chosen in light of changing abilities. Those with progressive MS and everyone affected by this process should be given support during this difficult time.

8

Gender-Related and Family Issues

Special Issues for Women

Multiple sclerosis (MS) is more common in women than in men—approximately 70 to 75 percent of people with MS are women. A number of issues are of special concern to women, including those related to the menstrual cycle, pregnancy, and menopause.

Menstruation

Women with MS often report temporary worsening of symptoms in the week before their menstrual period or during their period. Some more significantly disabled MS women, those with progressive disease, may actually experience a temporary worsening of their overall neurologic condition. Two recent studies of women with MS reported that MRI lesion activity may be related to hormonal fluctuations connected to the menstrual cycle. These studies await confirmation in larger numbers of patients.

Treatment with interferon beta, particularly in higher doses, can disrupt the menstrual cycle. There have been reports of abnormal Pap smears in women treated with glatiramer acetate, but this appears to be a coincidental finding.

Contraception and Fertility

There is no evidence that MS has a negative effect on the ability to conceive or has any negative effect on fertility. Many women with MS have children. In fact, some recent studies suggest that the long-term prognosis is better for women with MS who do have children.

With regard to MS medications, the use of cytotoxic immunosuppressive therapy can result in amenorrhea and even loss of fertility for women, and men's sperm counts may be affected. Patients need to be aware of this possibility before starting therapy. These drugs generally are reserved for people with more severe disease.

Pregnancy

Multiple sclerosis disease activity is less during pregnancy. The last trimester is particularly protective, with a 70 percent decrease in clinical relapses. This positive effect on MS appears to be due to a general immunosuppressive state during pregnancy, which becomes stronger in the later stages. Although there are no studies to confirm this, one would therefore expect that progressive MS might be under somewhat better control during pregnancy.

However, during the three months post partum there is a 70 percent increase in the clinical relapse rate, which basically cancels out the benefit of the latter part of pregnancy. It is a major concern that once the pregnancy ends, at least for a short period of time, there is actually an increase or worsening of MS disease activity. Again, this has never been studied specifically in progressive MS, but some anecdotal data suggest that women with secondary progressive MS may not do well following their pregnancies.

Recent studies suggest that breast-feeding may be protective, with a decrease in MS disease activity. The explanation for this is unclear, and further studies are needed to determine whether breast-feeding is truly protective.

At the current time, pregnancy and its effect on MS is under intensive research investigation to determine exactly what combination of factors may explain the protective effect. For the woman with progressive MS, who may be more significantly disabled, choices about pregnancy should be tempered with a realization that the degree of handicap that may be experienced after delivery may interfere with being able to take care of the child. Therefore, it is very important that a good support system be in place. In summary, there are no data indicating that pregnancy and birth ultimately have any long-term negative effects, although a reasonable expectation would be that there might be for several months a brief worsening of MS after giving birth.

Drug Therapies and Pregnancy

At the current time, it is generally recommended that women on MS disease-modifying therapies do not try to become pregnant and that they should stop disease-modifying therapy if they do become pregnant. It also has been recommended that women with MS who are breast-feeding should not be receiving disease-modifying therapy because the drugs may pass into their breast milk. These recommendations are based on U.S. Food and Drug Administration requirements. Data from animal models show that the interferon betas may cause abortion when given at a dose of approximately twice that used in MS. There is no evidence that these drugs cause damage to the fetus or that they are teratogenic (producing developmental malformations, or birth defects). Glatiramer acetate does not appear to have a negative effect either on pregnancy or on the fetus.

Basically for medicolegal reasons, rather than being based on clear medical evidence, most women with MS who are receiving disease-modifying therapies are using some form of contraception. They are taken off the medications if they become pregnant. In reality, a number of children have been born to women who have taken the disease-modifying therapies. It might be reasonable for a patient to continue on therapy if she is willing to take the risk. However, this decision should be made only after careful consideration and discussion with the physician.

Menopause

In most people, MS does not "burn out," and it is unrealistic to expect that the disease will improve over time. In fact, the reverse is true and MS can be expected to continue past menopause. Menopause does not appear to have any effect on MS, either positive or negative. However, this is an area in which very little formal research has been done. Anecdotal data indicate that MS symptoms that worsen, or appear to worsen, at the time of menopause may respond to hormone replacement therapy.

Hormone Replacement Therapy

Another area in which there are almost no formal studies involve hormone replacement therapy in women with MS. There does not appear to be any adverse effect of appropriate hormone replacement therapy on MS.

Sexual Dysfunction

Sexual dysfunction is one of the major symptoms of MS and a very common problem. It is estimated that 44 percent of women with MS are sexually inactive, and 40 to 80 percent report a variety of sexual problems, including decreased desire, problems with performance, problems with sensation or numbness in the vaginal area, pain during intercourse, decreased orgasms, decreased lubrication, and vaginismus (pain in the vagina). A variety of factors come into play with regard to sexual dysfunction in women with MS. *Primary* factors are those related to direct physical impairment from the neurologic deficits produced by MS. *Secondary* factors are those related to problems produced by the symptoms of MS, such as an inability to assume an appropriate position as a result of spasticity. *Tertiary* factors result from psychosocial issues, such as loss of a sense of self-worth and attractiveness.

The treatment of sexual dysfunction is based on the specific problems encountered. It may include counseling, discussion with the spouse, using glucocorticoids, lubrication, using alternative techniques such as a vibrator, and a redefinition of sexual activity to include a broader concept than penetration. It is very important in treating sexual dysfunction that your partner be involved in all counseling and discussions.

Miscellaneous Problems Associated with Beta Interferon

Rare problems associated with interferon betas have included alopecia (hair loss). Vascular headaches, which are more common in women in the first place, can be exacerbated by interferon beta. From a cosmetic point of view, subcutaneous injection of medications—more so with interferon beta than with glatiramer acetate—may cause injection-site reactions and skin lesions.

Special Issues for Men

Men are in the minority in the MS population, accounting for only 25 to 30 percent of those with the disease. However, approximately 50 percent of those with primary progressive disease are men. A number of gender-specific problems may arise in men with MS.

Sexual Dysfunction

Sexual dysfunction is common in men with MS, with up to 78 percent noting some form of erectile dysfunction. Other problems include decreased sexual activity and decreased libido. Therapies for erectile dysfunction include medications such as sildenafil (Viagra®). Side effects include flushing, headache, indigestion, hypertension, and visual difficulties. This medication is taken approximately one hour before arousal is expected. Sildenafil has basically supplanted the penile suppository MUSE® as well as the penile injection technique and Caverject. The treatment of sexual dysfunction is not only dependent on medication but also involves counseling, the involvement of your partner, and sometimes the use of glucocorticoids.

Contraception and Fertility

Contraception and fertility do not appear to be affected by MS, and many men with MS have fathered children. It is not necessary for men to worry about being on disease-modifying therapy, and no particular precaution needs to be taken. When immunosuppressive therapy (such as mitoxantrone) is used, there is a potential concern about effects on sperm count and fertility. Storage of donated sperm can be considered in such cases.

Prostate Function

As is true for all men, those with MS can develop prostate problems, including enlargement of the prostate and prostate cancer. This should be evaluated in routine medical examinations, which evaluate size of the prostate and, after a certain age, test for prostatic specific antigen, or PSA.

Parenting

The diagnosis of MS should not necessarily interrupt one's wishes or plans for parenthood. Multiple sclerosis may alter but should not affect the desire to experience the joys of parenting and the ability to provide children with the love and security they need. The best way to prepare for the years ahead with MS is to provide yourself with education and information about the disease along with the developmental needs of your children. The ultimate goal is for parents to achieve a level of comfort as an effective parenting team to maintain a sense of security despite the changes wrought by MS.

Because MS most often affects young people, it is common for people with the disease to have young children. It can be very difficult for children to deal with illness in their parents. It is important that children be aware of MS and informed about it. It should not be kept a secret. As they grow older, children need appropriate education and information about MS. Information about a parent's condition provides them with reassurance and reduces the fear of the unknown. It is often helpful for children to realize that they are not alone and that many others are in the same position, facing the same problems, and having to cope.

Accurate information about MS provides them with a vocabulary and creates boundaries around their fears. Children need to know that people rarely die of MS, that the disease is becoming increasingly treatable, and that they will not lose their parent. In younger children, education about MS helps to reduce and/or avoid the sense of self-blame or responsibility for a parent's condition. Children are observant and sense that something is not right in the family when their parents do not confide in them. By openly discussing an important issue, MS, the groundwork is laid for good parent–child communication for future issues that will arise as children grow and develop. Open lines of communication reduce secrecy and establish trust.

Research has demonstrated that children who have a parent with a disability or chronic illness are very much like those whose parents do not have major health problems. Children continue to develop despite added responsibilities as long as there are regular open lines of communication with their parents. As they become older, there may be a need for children to assume additional responsibilities in the home, responsibilities that are appropriate to their age and stage of development. Chores such as folding the laundry, setting the table, and supervising younger siblings may be added to children's tasks. Along with added responsibilities when a parent is disabled, children need time to be children. They need regular times to play, to participate in school activities, to be with friends, and to pursue sports or hobbies.

Parenting roles may need to be redefined for both men and women with MS. Fathers may not be able to play sports with their children; mothers may not be able to attend games and drive their children to special events. There should be no guilt on the parent's part, and the children can be taught that their parent can substitute with other activities and time spent together. It is important to emphasize parent–child communication and contact. Quality time spent together can take many forms; it may be as simple as reading a book together, watching a sports show, or going over homework.

It is also important to inform children's teachers about the diagnosis of MS. School is an important source of stability and self-confidence, and teachers are primary figures in the child's experiences. Once they are aware of MS, teachers can be helpful in gauging children's responses to the illness and to changes in the family. In addition, this awareness of the home situation will enable the teacher to be attentive to any changes in the child's school performance, social relationships, and emotional adjustment.

MS centers located throughout North America, the National Multiple Sclerosis Society, and local MS chapters sponsor special programs for children whose parents have MS. These programs can be extremely helpful in giving the children appropriate information, experts to talk to, and peers with whom to discuss problems and issues. Many chapters sponsor camp programs, family weekends, and counseling and support groups for children whose parents have MS.

Intimacy

Physicians and health care providers involved in the management of MS have tended to focus on its causes, symptoms, and treatment. They have not focused on issues of intimacy, which include but are not limited to the genital sexual response. It is critical that everyone with MS consider himself as a "whole" person with needs and desires for intimate relationships and that these issues be adequately addressed by the health care system. You have a right to a sexual life, and you should be assisted to probe and discover new and more effective ways to achieve satisfaction. Recognizing the limits imposed by the disease, it is important to accept and adapt to the strengths and limitations that it imposes rather than to restrict or cease your search for new means of sexual expression.

Because MS may have changed you in major ways and your sense of self as a man or woman may feel threatened, it is important to take stock of the situation. Asking the following questions may help: What has changed? What is the same? What can you still do or feel? What can you try to do to communicate your needs and desires to your loved one? Which sexual activities are no longer pleasant? Which ones continue to be pleasant?

The ability to achieve sexual satisfaction is the result of complex sets of physical and psychological interactions. A person must be comfortable in both the physical sense and the emotional sense to fully participate in moments of intimacy. This nurturing climate is of enormous help in reaching the maximum level of sexual potential. Communicating concerns to a loved one and/or to a health care provider often can identify the issues involved and separate the physiologic effects of MS from those that are psychological in nature. Patience and reciprocal caring can be of great value (both in and out of the bedroom) and should never be overlooked or underestimated.

Of Special Concern to Men

The ability to achieve and maintain an erection, have intercourse, and experience pleasurable sensations are important to all men. Multiple sclerosis may interfere with some of these important aspects of physical gratification and may cause problems for men and their sexual partners. Erection may be difficult to achieve and maintain, premature ejaculation may occur, and sometimes sensation is lost or diminished in the genital area. A frank discussion with a health care provider may yield some valuable information and some important interventions. Medications are available to treat impotence, and there are strategies for overcoming other physiologic changes.

Libido or sex drive usually is not affected by MS, but fatigue and depression may reduce sexual desire. Therefore, it is very important to treat and manage these symptoms (as discussed on Chapter 4). Many men have learned to include a variety of lovemaking techniques and not just to rely on intercourse as the only method of giving and receiving pleasure. Intimacy can consist of many ways of caring and communicating with one another.

Of Special Concern to Women

Many women with MS report vaginal dryness and problems with positioning due to bladder dysfunction or spasticity of one or both legs. A number of over-the-counter products are available for vaginal lubrication, and spasticity can be managed (as discussed in Chapter 4).

Explore New Options

As with other life activities, sexuality and intimacy are best achieved with an open mind and the ability to explore alternative options. You may discover and gain gratification in a wide variety of ways and at different levels of intensity. This is especially true when MS prevents you from self-expression in more "traditional" ways. Many people remain most comfortable with patterns that are familiar and have been developed over many years. With MS, these methods may no longer work. Therefore, a willingness to be flexible is likely to lead to a more enriching and gratifying sex life. Changes of position, body exploration, oral contact, and environmental adaptation may improve sexual function and increase opportunities for intimate moments.

Lack of sensation may also cause concern about orgasm. Orgasm is a very different experience for each individual; with MS, exacerbations or medications may produce difficulties. These natural variations do not mean decreased sexuality—these are *natural* variations and should be accepted as such. It is important to enjoy whatever pleasure you can give or receive at any given time.

Communicating Concerns

Although it is not unusual to experience difficulty in discussing sexual concerns with others, candid conversation often can facilitate a new awareness and consideration of sexual options and patterns that are more comfortable and work well. Sources of information about this topic are more readily available today in both the private and the public sectors. The National Multiple Sclerosis Society and the Coalition on Sexuality and Disability (122 E. 23 St., New York, NY 10010) are excellent resources about this topic. Although this information may be helpful, one should not view it as "gospel" about how to conduct one's personal life. Deciding how and when to conduct intimate relationships is and should remain a matter of wishes, tastes, and personal preferences.

Conclusion

We have tried to convey the sense that men and women have a right to express their sexuality and seek intimacy with understanding, joy, dignity, and positive feelings for self and others. Although MS may alter this ability somewhat, adjustments and considerations can and should be made to facilitate exploration and learning of new ways to find pleasure and to share pleasure with another. This fulfillment is natural and right for all people.

9

Taking Care: Prevent Complications and Stay Healthy

For anyone with a chronic disease, it becomes critically important to maximize health-promoting wellness factors (Table 9.1). People with multiple sclerosis (MS) can also develop other health problems, including hypertension, diabetes, ulcers, heart attacks, and cancer. They need to realize that not all new problems are due to MS and that regular medical checkups are as necessary for them as for anyone else.

The value of periodic screening of both well and chronically ill adults is well documented in today's health literature. It is the experience of most health care providers that a periodic meeting between a patient and a physician and/or nurse is of great benefit to screen for the risk of health care problems or to identify conditions that are affecting health status or quality of life. In the case of MS, underlying medical conditions can also alter the symptoms of MS and the person's functional status. Conditions to be screened include cardiovascular disease, including cholesterol, blood pressure, smoking, and stress; cancer (breast, prostate, testicular, and colorectal); osteoporosis; and safety (Table 9.2).

Women's Basic Health Care Screening

Women with MS are a particularly vulnerable group. They tend to have a large array of symptoms along with their primary and gynecologic needs.

Table 9.1 *Basic Health Considerations for People with Progressive Multiple Sclerosis*

- Do not smoke
- Follow a well-balanced diet
- Use alcohol with moderation
- Get enough sleep at night
- Institute a regular exercise program even if you do it from a wheelchair
- Try to maintain an optimal body weight
- Maintain hobbies and outside interests
- Keep a good mental attitude
- Use rest periods or naps to restore energy
- Get regular medical and dental checkups
- Women should get regular Pap smears, mammograms, and bone density tests to identify developing health problems
- Men should get regular prostate evaluations; those who use a wheelchair should also have regular bone density tests

Not surprisingly, a woman with MS often regards her neurologist as a primary care physician, who may or may not provide her with an adequate level of basic care. In general, women with MS, like women without health problems, require basic health care services in addition to neurologic follow-up.

A general and complete physical examination should be performed for women between the ages of 40 to 50 at least every three years. Between 50 and 65 years the recommendation increases to an examination every second year and after age 65 to an annual examination. The examination should include cancer screening in the form of a Pap smear, a clinical breast examination to identify potential malignancies, and routine laboratory tests as well as an electrocardiogram and a chest X-ray. A rectal examination is recommended after the age of 40, and a stool (fecal material) examination for blood and endoscopy (examination of the large intestine) should be performed after the age of 50 (Table 9.2).

Men's Basic Health Care Screening

Men should follow similar guidelines for full medical checkups. Because of the high risk of cardiovascular disease in men between 50 and 60 years, it is very important to have a baseline electrocardiogram and blood work initially at age 40 and then on a regular basis thereafter. Testicular cancer is a common problem in young men and regular self-examination is recommended; prostate cancer is frequently encountered in the aging male pop-

Table 9.2 *Guidelines for Adult Screening*

Procedure	Women <50	Women 50–64	Women >65	Men <50	Men 50–64	Men >65
Screening						
Blood pressure	Annually	Annually	Annually	Annually	Annually	Annually
Cholesterol	Once	Every 5 yrs.	Every 5 yrs.	Once	Every 5 yrs.	Every 5 yrs.
Fecal blood	—	Annually	Annually	—	Annually	Annually
Sigmoidoscopy	—	Every 5–10 yrs.	Every 5–10 yrs.	—	Every 5–10 yrs.	Every 5–10 yrs.
CBE	Annually after 40	Annually	Annually			
Mammography		Every 1–2 yrs.	Every 1–2 yrs. to 75			
Pap	Every 3 yrs. if sex active	Every 3 yrs. if sex active	Every 3 yrs. to 75			
Vision			Annually			Annually
Hearing		Every 5 yrs.			Every 5 yrs.	
PPD	Patient at risk	Patient at risk	Patient at risk			
Immunizations						
Td	Every 10 yrs.	Every 10 yrs.	Every 10 yrs.	Every 10 yrs.	Every 10 yrs.	Every 10 yrs.
Influenza	Patient at risk (annually)	Patient at risk (annually)	Annually	Annually	Annually	Annually
Pneumococcal	Patient at risk (once)	Patient at risk (once)	Once	Patient at risk (once)	Patient at risk (once)	Once
Annual Counseling						
Smoking	+	+	+	+	+	+
Exercise	+	+	+	+	+	+
Diet						
Calcium Intake	+	+	+			
Fat			+			+
Sex Education	+	+	+	+	+	+
Depression			+			+
Injury Prevention			+			+
Alcohol/Driving	+	+	+	+	+	+

CBE, clinical breast examination; PPD, purified protein derivative; Td, tetanus = diphtheria.

ulation. A digital rectal examination should be performed annually but may not be as sensitive as a simple blood test. Prostatic specific antigen (PSA) testing is recommended after the age of 40 and regularly thereafter to screen for prostate cancer.

Osteoporosis

An area of preventive care of concern to both men and women is the risk of osteoporosis. Osteoporosis is a progressive disorder of bone mass loss that can lead to serious problems such as bodily deformity (loss of height, rounding of the back, changes in body stature), pain, and low-impact fracture. Although most people associate this problem primarily with women, everyone with MS is at particular risk because of the tendency to decreased weight bearing and the frequent use of steroids. In addition, other risk factors include being a Caucasian woman of small frame, genetic factors (a family history of osteoporosis), environmental factors (cigarette and alcohol use), a calcium-poor diet, and inadequate sun exposure.

Both women and men should have bone mineral density testing, the most sensitive measure for evaluating osteoporosis status. Risk factors that can be modified include the elimination of cigarettes and alcohol, maintenance of normal body weight, and vigilant attention to the prevention of falls. People who are not involved in any exercise should engage in a program to promote bone rebuilding, either actively or passively. In menopausal women, hormone replacement therapy may be indicated after evaluation by a gynecologist in collaboration with the primary care physician or neurologist. Other protective treatment includes calcium supplementation, usually in a dose of 1,000 mg per day for premenopausal women and 1,500 mg per day for postmenopausal women. A daily multivitamin will facilitate absorption of calcium into the blood stream.

Dental Care

Any type of infection will trigger MS symptoms. This includes dental problems such as caries or periodontal disease. It is important to see a dentist at least annually, to avoid frequent snacks or sugar-containing foods, and to brush your teeth with fluoridated toothpaste twice a day. Flossing is also advisable to reduce the accumulation of food at the gum margins or between the teeth.

Diet and Nutrition

Your body needs about 40 different nutrients to stay healthy, including vitamins, minerals, protein, carbohydrates, fats (in limited quantity), and water. No single food item can supply all the essential nutrients your body needs. The U.S. Department of Agriculture has stated that a well-balanced diet should consist primarily of complex carbohydrates, which are contained in breads, cereals, fruits, vegetables, legumes, nuts, and seeds (Figure 9.1). Food containing fat and simple sugars should be limited. Use herbs and spices rather than salt to season your food. Avoid too many sweets, which, as stated earlier, can cause tooth decay and result in weight gain. Drink alcohol only in moderation because alcohol is high in calories and low in nutrition.

To reduce fat and cholesterol intake, choose lean meat, fish, poultry, dry beans, and peas; moderate the number of eggs and organ meats you eat; limit your intake of butter, cream, shortening, coconut oil, and foods made with these products; trim excess fat from meats; broil, bake, or boil food rather than fry; and read labels carefully.

It is important to drink an adequate amount of fluids to maintain all bodily functions. Fluids provide the lubrication that helps you swallow and keeps your tissues hydrated. They form waste products and body fluids such as blood, lymph, and perspiration. They also help retain moisture in the skin, hair, and nails. Inadequate fluid intake can contribute to constipation, urinary tract infection, and skin breakdown. A minimum of eight glasses of fluids should be drunk daily and can be obtained indirectly by eating gelatin-based desserts and other foods make from liquids.

An adequate intake of food and fluids fuels the body for all activities of daily living and is an important key to wellness.

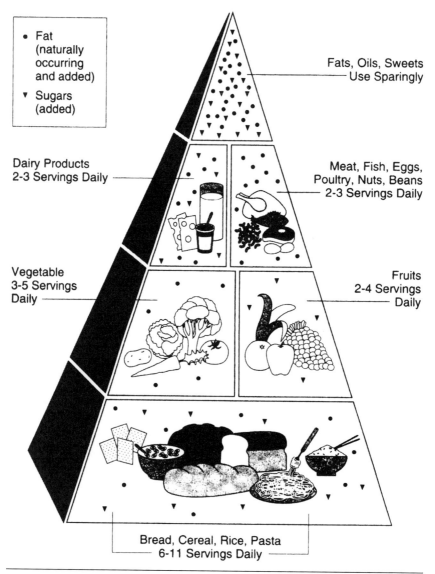

Figure 9.1   *A Guide to Daily Food Choices*
Source: U.S. Department of Agriculture/U.S. Department of health and Human Services

A

Additional Readings

NOTE: *Your local chapter of the National Multiple Sclerosis Society has a complete collection of booklets and articles about all aspects of MS research, treatments, and management. Call 1-800-FIGHT MS to be connected to the chapter nearest you. Chapter personnel are available to answer your questions and send you information on any MS-related topics that are of interest to you.*

General Reference
Kalb RC. (1998). *Multiple Sclerosis: A Guide for Families.* New York: Demos Medical Publishing.

Chapter 3. Disease-Modifying Therapy
Giffels JJ. (1996). *Clinical Trials: What You Should Know Before Volunteering to Be a Research Subject.* New York: Demos.

Chapter 4. Managing the Symptoms of Progressive Multiple Sclerosis
Polman CH, Thompson AJ, Murray, TJ, McDonald WI. (2001) *Multiple Sclerosis: The Guide to Treatment and Management,* 5th ed. New York: Demos Medical Publishing.

Schapiro RT. (1998). *Symptom Management in Multiple Sclerosis* (3rd ed.). New York: Demos Medical Publishing.

Adapted from Kalb RC, *Multiple Sclerosis: The Questions You Have—The Answers You Need,* 2nd ed. New York: Demos Medical Publishing, 2000.

Chapter 5. Facing the Challenge of Worsening Multiple Sclerosis: Tools for the Transition

Lunt S. (1982). *A Handbook for the Disabled: Ideas and Inventions for Easier Living*. New York: Scribners.

Chapter 6. Increasing Disability: Social and Economic Issues

Cooper L. (2001). *Insurance Solutions: Plan Well, Live Better—A Workbook for People with a Chronic Disease or Disability*. New York: Demos Medical Publishing.

Mendelsohn SB. (1996). *Tax Options and Strategies for People with Disabilities*, 2nd ed. New York: Demos.

Perkins L, Perkins S. (1999). *Multiple Sclerosis: Your Legal Rights*, 2nd ed. New York: Demos Medical Publishing.

Resources for Rehabilitation (1993a). *Meeting the Needs of Employees with Disabilities*. Lexington, MA: Resources for Rehabilitation.

Rumrill PD, Jr. (ed.). (1996). *Employment Issues and Multiple Sclerosis*. New York: Demos.

Stolman MD. (1994). *A Guide to Legal Rights for People with Disabilities*. New York: Demos.

Chapter 7. Coping with Disease Progression

Cooke M, Putman E. (1996). *Ways You Can Help: Creative, Practical Suggestions for Family and Friends of Patients and Caregivers*. New York: Warner Books.

Halligan F. (1995). *The Art of Coping*. New York: Crossroad.

Kalb RC. (1998). *Multiple Sclerosis: A Guide for Families*. Demos Medical Publishing.

Koplowitz A, Celizic M. (1997). *The Winning Spirit: Lessons Learned in Last Place*. New York: Doubleday.

LeMaistre J. (1994). *Beyond Rage: Mastering Unavoidable Health Changes*. Dillon, CO: Alpine Guild.

Peterman Schwarz S. (1999). *300 Tips for Making Life with Multiple Sclerosis Easier*. New York: Demos Medical Publishing.

Wells SM. (1998). *A Delicate Balance: Living Successfully with Chronic Illness*. New York: Plenum Press.

Chapter 8. Gender-Related and Family Issues

Cristall B. (1992). *Coping When a Parent Has Multiple Sclerosis.* New York: Rosen Publishing [written for teens].

Kalb RC. (1998). *Multiple Sclerosis: A Guide for Families.* Demos Medical Publishing.

Kroll K, Klein EL. (1995). *Enabling Romance: A Guide to Love, Sex, and Relationships for the Disabled.* Bethesda, MD: Woodbine House.

Sherkin-Langer F. (1995). *When Mommy Is Sick.* St. Louis: Fern Publications (P.O. Box 16893, St. Louis, MO 63105; fax: 314-994-0052. [Recommended for children ages 2–8].

Strong M. (1997). *For the Well Spouse of the Chronically Ill,* 3rd rev. Mainstay, NY: Little, Brown.

Wright LM, Leahey M. (1987). *Families and Chronic Illness.* Philadelphia: Spring House.

Chapter 9. Taking Care: Prevent Complications and Stay Healthy

Bowling AC. (2001). *Alternative Medicine and Multiple Sclerosis.* New York: Demos Medical Publishing.

Holland N, Halper J. (eds.). (1998). *Multiple Sclerosis: A Self-Care Guide to Wellness.* Washington, DC: Paralyzed Veterans of America.

Kraft GH, Catanzaro M. (2000). *Living with Multiple Sclerosis: A Wellness Approach,* 2nd ed. New York: Demos Medical Publishing.

B

Resources

National Multiple Sclerosis Society (NMSS) (733 Third Avenue, New York, NY 10017; tel: 800-FIGHT MS; Internet: www.nmss.org). The NMSS is a nonprofit organization that supports national and international research into the prevention, cure, and treatment of MS. The Society's goals include provision of nationwide services to assist people with MS and their families, and provision of information to those with MS, their families, professionals, and the public. The programs and services of the Society promote knowledge, health, and independence while providing education and emotional support:

- Toll-free access to your local chapter by selecting the option one at 800-FIGHT MS.
- Internet web site with updated information about treatments, current research, and programs (http://www,nmss.org); local home page in many areas.
- Knowledge Is Power self-study program (serial mailings) for people newly diagnosed with MS and their families, available through most chapters.
- Moving Forward, an on-line education series for people newly diagnosed with MS and their families, available on the NMSS web site.

Printed materials available on a variety of topics from your local chapter.

- Educational programs on various topics throughout the year, provided through your local chapter
- Annual national teleconference at over 500 sites throughout the United States; call your chapter for the location nearest you
- Swimming and other exercise programs sponsored or co-sponsored by some chapters, or referral to existing programs in the community
- Wellness programs in some chapters

Multiple Sclerosis Society of Canada (250 Bloor Street East, Suite 1000, Toronto, Ontario M4W 3P9, Canada; tel: 416-922-6065; in Canada: 800-268-7582; Internet: www.mssoc.ca). A national organization that funds research, promotes public education, and produces publications in both English and French. They provide an "ASK MS Information System" database of articles on a wide variety of topics including treatment, research, and social services. Regional divisions and chapters are located throughout Canada.

Consortium of Multiple Sclerosis Centers (CMSC) (c/o Gimbel MS Center at Holy Name Hospital, 718 Teaneck Road, Teaneck, NJ 07666; tel: 201-837-0727; Internet: www.mscare.org). The CMSC is made up of numerous MS centers throughout the United States and Canada. The Consortium's mission is to disseminate information to clinicians, increase resources and opportunities for research, and advance the standard of care for multiple sclerosis. The CMSC is a multidisciplinary organization, bringing together health care professionals from many fields involved in MS patient care.

Department of Veterans Affairs (VA) (810 Vermont Avenue, N.W., Washington, D.C. 20420; tel: 202-273-5400; Internet: www.va.org). The VA provides a wide range of benefits and services to those who have served in the armed forces, their dependents, beneficiaries of deceased veterans, and dependent children of veterans with severe disabilities.

Paralyzed Veterans of America (PVA) (801 Eighteenth Street N.W., Washington, D.C. 20006; tel: 800-424-8200; Internet: www.pva.org). PVA is a national information and advocacy agency working to restore function and quality of life for veterans with spinal cord dysfunction. It supports and funds education and research and has a national advocacy program that focuses on accessibility issues. PVA publishes brochures on many issues related to rehabilitation.

Social Security Administration (6401 Security Boulevard, Baltimore, MD 21235; tel: 800-772-1213; Internet: www.ssa.gov). To apply for social security benefits based on disability, call this office or visit your local social security branch office. The Office of Disability within the Social Security

Administration publishes a free brochure entitled "Social Security Regulations: Rules for Determining Disability and Blindness."

Through the Looking Glass: National Research and Training Center on Families of Adults with Disabilities (2198 Sixth Street, Suite 100, Berkeley, CA 94710; tel: 510-848-4445; 800-644-2666; Internet: www.lookingglass.org).

Electronic Information Sources

There are many sources of information available free through the Internet on the World Wide Web. If you are an experienced "net surfer," switch to your favorite search facility and enter the key words "MS" or "multiple sclerosis." This will generally give you a listing of dozens of web sites that pertain to MS. Keep in mind, however, that the World Wide Web is a free and open medium; while many of the web sites have excellent and useful information, others may contain highly unusual and inaccurate information. Following is a list of just a few of many MS sites available through the Internet. Each of these will provide links to other sites.

ABLEDATA
Information on Assistive Technology
http://www.abledata.com/

Allsup, Inc
Assists Individuals Applying for Social Security Disability Benefits
http://www.allsupinc.com/

Apple Computer Disability Resources
http://www.apple.com/education/k12/disability/

The Ares-Serono Group/Rebif
http://www.serono.com/ms/

Berlex/Betaseron
http://www.betaseron.com/

Biogen/Avonex
http://www.biogen.com/

CLAMS—Computer Literate Advocates for Multiple Sclerosis
http://www.clams.org/

The Consortium of Multiple Sclerosis Centers
http://www.mscare.org/

IBM Special Needs Systems
http://www.austin.ibm.com/sns/

Infosci
Selected Links on MS
http://www.infosci.org/

International Federation of Multiple Sclerosis Societies/The World of
     Multiple Sclerosis
http://www.nmss.org/

The International Journal of MS Care
http://www.mscare.com/

Medicare Information
http://www.hcfa.gov/medicare/medicare.htm

Microsoft Accessibility Technology for Everyone
http://www.microsoft.com/enable/

The Multiple Sclerosis Society of Canada
http://www.mssoc.ca/

The National Family Caregivers Association
http://www.nfcacares.org/

The National Multiple Sclerosis Society
http://www.nmss.org/

Teva Marion Partners/Copaxone
http://www.tevamarionpartners.com/

Adapted from Kalb RC, *Multiple Sclerosis: The Questions You Have—The Answers
     You Need*, 2nd ed. New York: Demos Medical Publishing, 2000.

Index

Note: Boldface numbers indicate illustrations; italic *(t)* indicates a table.

Demos Medical Publishing, Inc. publishes numerous books on multiple sclerosis. These include:

Alternative Medicine and Multiple Sclerosis
Allen C. Bowling

Multiple Sclerosis: A Guide for the Newly Diagnosed
Nancy J. Holland, T. Jock Murray, and Stephen C. Reingold

Multiple Sclerosis: The Questions You Have—The Answers You Need,
2nd edition
Rosalind C. Kalb

Multiple Sclerosis: A Guide for Families
Rosalind C. Kalb

Multiple Sclerosis: Your Legal Rights, 2nd edition
Lanny E. Perkins and Sara D. Perkins

300 Tips for Making Life with Multiple Sclerosis Easier
Shelley Peterman Schwarz

Multiple Sclerosis: The Guide to Treatment and Management, 5th edition
Chris H. Polman, Alan J. Thompson,
T. Jock Murray, and W. Ian McDonald

Employment Issues in Multiple Sclerosis
Phillip D. Rumrill, Jr.

Symptom Management in Multiple Sclerosis, 3rd edition
Randall T. Schapiro

To receive additional information on these or any of our other titles,
call our toll-free number:
(800) 532-8663

Demos Medical Publishing, Inc.
386 Park Avenue South
New York, NY 10016
Phone (212) 683-0072
Fax (212) 683-0118
E-mail: orderdept@demospub.com
Website: demosmedpub.com

CLAYTON-LIBERTY TWP LIBRARY
Clayton, IN 46118